MARTIN

for
MARTIN
a boy who grew up

CONTENTS

Introduction

I sat in the place where I take all my sorrow. Hard shell of a woman I used to be. The hovering shadow of death had descended, obliterating all life in me. Such women as I, deprived of a person around whom the whole world revolves, fall easily into faithlessness and despair.

My mind wept, inside the shell, as it had been doing daily for weeks. I felt beside me a wheelchair padded with blankets, containing a muffled child. He sat, meekly passive, patient and resigned. He had all he wanted out of life, just to sit there in the presence he knew, being with me.

But he wasn't there. I looked and the aisle was empty, gaping wide. Whatever lay beyond that long, dreamless sleep for him, I was alone.

The sword of division fell again, the

wound renewed. I gave myself to the mourning as it bled.

Then out from the air, above and ahead, a bright lively voice emerged. 'Write about me,' it said.

The message, urgent and alert, pierced the shell, sending an arrow to the soul. My mind now saw a day early in Summer, outside the church. We'd been on a walk and had paused on the way back, as was our habit.

'One day,' I told him flatly, parking the wheelchair so it wouldn't run, 'I'm going to write a book!'

It was meant as an exasperated comment on life, the heat, the hectic pace, the switchback, and the hefty exercise that wretched chair could be.

'Oh yes,' he responded, as always to anything new, 'write about me.'

I looked at him, as I passed to go inside. A story indeed. 'Yes I will,' I promised. 'I'll write about you.'

It was an idea. With genuine humility, he loved publicity, unknowing the limelight it drew. My doing anything was something we shared. It was sheer love to publicise our partnership. Anything, even to mounting Everest with that chair, I would do to please him.

But inside the church, the woman in me lurched. What time had I, what freedom of mind, what heart, to tackle a book? We didn't know, either one of us, and nor did any man, what the end was to be.

Now I have the time; a little space in a life that can never be easy. I know the end. He has reminded me of my promise; 'Write about me.' Over and over again I have rejected those words, in a ruthless agony. Re-tread that road? Revive that ordeal? No! I must forget.

But the spirit went on, till I gave in. He would not leave me be. Relentless in pursuit, the excited spirit; 'Write about me.'

So for him I take the pick to frozen memory, fearful of what it may reveal. For him I grope for courage to journey the Valley of the Shadow, just once again.

My baby, my hero, my saint and my beloved son, whom God took aside and made into a man.

CHAPTER 1

The boy

He was born at home, on the seventeenth of October, the fifth child of the family. He kept everybody waiting.

Long labour was my norm. A neighbour who had given up her night's sleep to witness the miracle of birth left, hours before it occurred. Her patience exceeded mine.

We had just reached the point of no return when the plan for home confinement had to be abandoned. The doctor went to telephone to arrange admission to hospital, and was half way down the stairs when the midwife called him up again. As though he knew, Martin Gerard had decided to arrive.

The home he was born into was not happy, at least not for me. Just a few months before, I too had reached a point of crisis, uncertain whether to go or stay. Was it better for the children to keep this unit as it was, or should they be removed from the atmosphere, and a new home set up elsewhere now? Would it uproot and bruise them so radically as to change their lives? Would the conflict, hidden but deep, do them irreparable harm?

Long weeks I thrashed about, tearing my mind, analysing conscience, only to decide at last the sacrifice must be made. My own life and my personal feelings must come second to the children and their security. I buried myself in their need and determined to make it work.

Martin gave me fresh incentive but also added to the strain. A small, puny infant, he immediately fell victim to an autumn germ and was put on to antibiotics. It was weeks before I knew a night's sleep or any semblance of domestic order. By the time a relative offered to take him, to give me relief, I was really at breaking point. I packed him on the bus, carrycot and all, and didn't care if I never saw him again.

The apathy of fagitue.

A week later, well slept and missing him unbearably, I had him returned. He recovered, filled out, grew and responded to my devotion.

The most lovable thing about him was his smile; early, sweet and quite sublime. It radiated everything. I only had to look at him, sometimes, to feel it all worthwhile. As a toddler he loved to cuddle up beside me and be 'one' with me, his nature once more merged into mine. Not saying anything. Not moving. Communicating love. It is an age for making foundations and the bond between us was sound.

A loving, enquiring child, he seemed to sense my sorrow and my need of him. A dead marriage is a failed relationship; for me, a failed vocation. He clung to me and gave it meaning. It had, after all, given me him. We were all right, we two, so long as we had each other. His baby smile went right through my eyes and took root in my soul.

Later on two more babies came, both

boys. Martin merged happily into the team. No momma's boy, and no weakling now, he gave himself to all the joys of a boy. He swung on the swing, got wet in water, rode anything that moved and ate anything that didn't eat him first. When television came to the home, he thrilled to it and used it, with every facet of his keen, active, mind.

When he was clean, he had an air of refined gentleness that appealed. It was getting and keeping him that way that was the difficulty. Hypersensitive and averse to washing, he squirmed and wriggled till I couldn't site the cloth.

'For pity's sake, stand *still,'* I'd yell at him, the others queuing for their turn.

'I can't,' miserably, in genuine martyrdom.

'Look,' I suggested practically, 'offer it up for the holy souls. Get somebody out of Purgatory.'

At that he set his muscle, under his mind. He stood stiff, hands clasped tight behind his waist, and suffered nobly for the cause.

He did master it, in time. But he never enjoyed it.

He was a good boy, in the sense of being obedient, not without mischief or fun. Once I had explained to him the difference between right and wrong, in his daily living, he simply obeyed. Only when he didn't know did he go astray. He was eager to learn.

Once, he was involved in the stealing of sweets from a corner shop; the gay habit of companions. His honest soul went through the torment of Hell. It was completely out of character.

Sternly I explained to him the consequences of petty crime and the loss of status in the criminal. He apologised and was punished, and made amends. I assured him that he was forgiven. But he clung to me in taut anguish, unable to forget. 'I'll never do it again Mam. Never.'

He learned easily.

He was a clever child; quick, lively, with a bright turn of wit and amazing energy. Late nights never bothered him as they slowed me. School reports revealed him as hard-working, helpful and pleasant. He was usually top of his Form. Study was effortless, examination painless. Success left him pleased but unspoiled. There was no trace of conceited bragging, or silly vanity.

Religion he took for granted and enjoyed. He loved to be in church, lit his candles intently and studiously prayed. Christ was a man and a big hero. Mary was a real lady. God could do anything, even the impossible, and was always reachable.

At home in his Father's house, he was not averse to high spirits. Piously praying in the sacred few minutes after my Communion during Mass, I was surprised to hear a fierce whisper in my ear, 'What's red and lies upside down in the gutter?' 'I don't know,' curiously. 'What?'. He giggled 'A dead bus'.

But on the bleak April day he made his own First Communion, his joy and pride went deep. He turned in the pew and sent to me, his sole parent, a telegraphic, wise, angelic smile. He was beginning a new relationship with God and the man from Nazareth; something we could share.

How seriously he took his faith I was still unaware, until one day I was collecting material for an article on boys and vocations to the priesthood.

'The Church needs 300,000 priests,' I threw out to the family casually. 'Any offers?'

I knew what to expect. Hard comment came like hail.

'It's boring...

'You get no peace...

'You're always dashing about, seeing sick people...

'I want to be an electrician.'

And from the eldest, the understatement of the year, 'It doesn't pay very well.'

Martin alone said firmly, undaunted by their cynicism, 'I want to be a priest.'

I silenced the others and asked carefully, 'Why Martin?'

'Because I want to be holy.'

Hoots all round.

We ignored them.

'And what else?', gently.

'Because I love God.' He thought hard and decided, 'I want to hold God. In my hands.'

He was eight years old; a little early to bother the Bishop. A few weeks later he began to have trouble with is leg.

CHAPTER 2

My leg hurts

Martin loved school, but he loved home even more, and was an expert at nine-o-clock pains. That's the kind that cripple in the early morning but disappear when the school bell rings. It was nothing to find him slow or missing at breakfast time, but I knew the signs. He was quickly found, spruced up and despatched, with an egg sandwich and a lecture on St George.

No bright lad in his right mind gets a pain like that on a Saturday, and it was a weekend when he complained of his leg.

It seemed tense and tender, difficult to move, between his right hip and knee. Sunday the pain was still there, nagging like a toothache. He was relieved when I said he needn't bother to go to Mass.

He spent the day resting on the settee with a heap of light reading and meals-on-wheels. So long as he was still, he was happy and content. When he got up to go to the toilet, he limped. It was obvious he couldn't use the leg normally.

I decided he had probably pulled a muscle and gave him a week off school. It was a long walk there and back. Better pamper the leg now and get it thoroughly fit.

At the end of the week he didn't really want to go back, but the nurse in me felt him ready for exercise after the period of rest. I was under severe duress myself, domestically. Among seven children a leg-pull is nothing dramatic. It wore off, he went back, and it was forgotten.

A few weeks later, it struck again. He seemed apologetic. There was no reason; no injury, no boisterious activity; nothing to be seen. It simply weakened and was left strained.

Never a reckless and dangerously head-strong boy where activity was concerned, he was now crying off school sport, and outdoor games. When the others dashed around the streets, he seemed now to prefer to be with me. He didn't follow me around, but simply sat quiet, doing something with hands instead of limbs, or watching television.

He was still finely built, ever ready for meals, but his appetite had lost its ferocity. At times it was a problem pleasing it. I adapted, and found ways of giving him only what he wanted, without catching the attention of the others. No sense preparing him food to waste.

Then he developed a most irritating and frustrating habit. When we were all out together, as happened frequently with so much shopping, instead of customarily streaking on ahead, Martin began lagging behind. Slower and slower he walked. Time after time, forging on with the push-chair leading the brood, enough on my mind to weigh down the moon, I'd look back to find him so far back he held up the crocodile.

'Come on love,' I'd urge him, time at a premium. 'What's wrong with you?'

He didn't seem to know. He just smiled.

So eventually he came to be left at home, by a choice that was mutual, unless I was going out alone. On those occasions, he was ready with alacrity. We held hands, and suited my pace to his, which was soothing to me. We forgot the life that was dragging us both by the heels, and enjoyed each other's company.

About every six weeks, that pain came again and had him on the settee. He wouldn't admit to illness and absolutely refused to stay in bed. I tried massage and liniment. I tried exercise. I rested it, warmed it, cooled it, bathed it, bandaged it; nothing worked. The relentless beat of its occurrence was giving me concern. Still he insisted it wasn't bad enough to warrant a doctor. A week or so, and he was back at school.

At this stage the disastrous and quite tragic relationship between his father and myself made it impossible for us to live under the same roof. I had for some time been seeking and taking advice of solicitors, priests, marriage counsellor and probation officer. The children were showing positive signs of neurosis; nightmares and sleep-walking and fear. Martin's dread of his father's presence was showing in his face, affecting his voice. I was in a state of perpetual depression. It could not go on.

I had made enquiries about quietly setting up a separate home. I had no money of my own, but was assured that, until I could find work, we would be maintained by the State. It was a deeply revolting procedure for me, with my ideals of marriage and family life, but reality has to be seen. Things had come to dangerous deadlock. It was, for us, the only solution.

His parents' affairs are not relevant to Martin, except in that they drew us closer together. He suffered more than the others; uniquely in my suffering. Child though he was, his understanding was more complete, his concern more obvious, his feelings more unselfish, and his compassion more generous than in all the rest together.

Sufficient to say that the marriage blew up in our faces one Friday night in May when Martin was nine. He spent the night in my bed, praying, while I packed the cases. We left the next morning, myself and the four youngest children, by taxi to the only sanctuary I knew; a convent of the Sisters of Nazareth where I was already known.

We were homeless and penniless, the roots of our past completely lifted out. We had to find a space to recover, then a safe place to put them down again and start a new life.

CHAPTER 3

Don't leave me

Martin was in his natural element, playing with the children at the Home run by the nuns. The grounds were wide and full of facilities to distract a juvenile. He was quite happy to stay behind. After a meal, I went out to seek accommodation.

It was Whitsun; a Bank Holiday. All the Welfare offices were closed. Advertisements abounded, however, in local shop windows; flats, bed-sitters and rooms. It wouldn't take me long, I felt. We'd soon be settled. I rather enjoyed the challenge, aside from the prospect, of a new home and life. At least I was free to attend to the family needs without interference, which was new for me.

It was dark before I returned, sore and defeated. The children, watching television, were tired and strained. Playing without me was one thing. Ending a day among strangers, unknowing the time of my return, was a cause for acute anxiety.

Under all those shope notices ought to have been printed in letters of red 'NO CHILDREN'. Places at a price, were available for me. Nobody would have a family at all.

The Sisters nobly fixed us up with beds, meals, and a visitor's room which allowed us a little privacy. We were still a family.

But at the end of four days, trailing streets, touring offices, talking myself dry, I was forced to realise, we weren't going to be able to stay that way. The State would not begin to maintain us until I had an address. I couldn't stay at the convent indefinitely. Looking after the young ones myself; washing, feeding and taking them out, preserving the mother-child relationship and the unit we were, I could not follow the housing trail and find us a home. There were also the three eldest, back where we had left, in varying emotional states. I was their mother too.

Distraught and exhausted, in a state of despair, I went to the priest who ran the Diocesan Rescue Society and fell on his mercy. He agreed to take the children, and let them stay where they were, provided I set myself to the task of making a home for them. I was insulted that he should even suspect me of doing otherwise, but later on came to realise his need for caution.

I had left the children playing in a nearby Dene, while I made the arrangements. They had no idea what I was doing. It was a lovely day, warm and serene; the atmosphere of holiday abandon greeted me. Only after an ice-cream and a drink did I tell them the news. 'You're going to stay with the Sisters a while, until I find a house.'

Faces fell. The little one, just three, did an unconcerned somersault in the grass. I explained to the others that I could get around a lot faster, and find us a home more rapidly, if I hadn't them to see to.

They couldn't stay on holiday indefinitely. They had to go to school. It would be easier from there, among new friends. I emphasised the temporary nature of it and assured them 'It won't be long.'

We walked back to the Home, a new gloom come down to cloud us as a group. Sullen silence from them denoted confusion, inability to understand. Too much by far, had already hit such vulnerable ages as twelve and five. I knew well the outcome of mother-deprivation. All I had done, at not little cost, since the first child was born, to ensure their security. Now here it was threatened again.

Brightly I tried to cheer them, over my own agony. This was a contingency I had not even remotely contemplated. Such things happen to other people. I thought of all their need for me, and my need for them. Bereft of all I had known and loved and built over the years, I needed them around me. We were close as refugees, my motherlove intensified. As much as I was their security, it seemed, they were mine.

The little one had been badly frightened

as an infant, he was terrified of running water. What happened when his bath-time came and he screamed for me?

I turned my tear-filled eyes to forget, and there he was, Martin as usual lagging behind. But this time tears flooded his eyes, ran fast down his face and dripped soulfully on to his lapels. I ran back and grabbed him to me, silent and hard.

'You can't leave, *me,*' he sobbed, racked at the very idea. 'Don't leave me.'

The sword went clear through to my spine. Of all the little ones, this spindly scrap was bleeding me. The coat I'd bought a year before was still too big. It magnified his need. He wanted what I couldn't give and I needed him.

So I straightened up and gave him a dose of what God had given me over the years. 'Come on now. Stop being a baby. We have to be very brave. We have a war to fight and we're going to win. They're not going to keep us apart.' I sniffed. 'We look stupid. I'll make you a deal. You stop crying and so will I.'

He sniffed to match. The long cuff of

his coat back-handed his eyes, streaking his cheeks. He held my hand, tight as a vice, and we walked up after the others.

'I wanted to come with *you,*' be bleated plaintively, weakening again. 'Can't I come with you?'

He couldn't. I couldn't tell him, because it could only increase instability; I didn't know where I was going.

I shook my head. 'I'll make you a promise,' I consoled. 'I'll come and see you every day. I'll bring you your comics. And as soon as I find a place where there's room for you, I'll bring you out. Even if I can't take the others. You'll be first.'

It seemed to appease.

I took them all in, gave them tea, and sent them out to play. Then I had a long talk with Reverend Mother.

That night they were registered, moved out of our room and into the dormitories; and issued with clothes. They looked strange, unsure of themselves, attempting to adapt to this wider family.

The youngest was separated from the

rest and put in a different corridor.I bathed him, loving him every minute, put him in his new bed and sat with him till he was asleep. I dared not imagine his reaction in the morning when he woke to find me gone.

I packed a case with what I needed, from the little we had brought. I said goodnight to the others, giving each a special hug, and reminding them I'd see them tomorrow.

My heart wrenched off its hinges, I trod wearily down the long, winding drive, through the iron gates and out into life alone.

CHAPTER 4

Apart

It was not my intention, at this stage, to go out to work. The flexible arrangement I had with the nuns meant I still did a lot for the children. My mother, a widow living alone, was unwell and needing our relationship. The older children were meeting me regularly and had to be supervised. My free hours I needed for touring estate agents, following up advertisements, finding us a home.

But it became obvious that, however frugally I lived, I could not depend on that State for security. I was classed as a single woman. The family allowances had been taken from me. School uniform accounts had to be paid. With necessities, fares, outings to keep us together, the five pounds a week I received from Social

Security was gone in three days.

That apart, a rented house the size we required, I now knew, was not likely to materialise. My only hope was in the long term project of raising a deposit, obtaining a mortgage and buying a house of our own.

How long that was going to take I dared not analyse. I'm not good at figures. I just knew the impetus to make a start. I had to find employment where I could earn enough to live decently, keep the children happy, and also save.

I had had some little success with writing; freelance fiction and social reporting. But as a means of making a living it is unreliable. A full-time writer needs a free mind, contacts and regular commissions. Too often hard labour results in rude, impersonal refusal without explanation. I hadn't time for that.

I was also doing a little television, by appointment, and explored the field there. At my age, with my ties, and no union membership, the prospects were nil.

That left me with nursing, for which I was trained and qualified. Hospital days were far behind, but I had recently been caring for terminal cancer cases, odd nights. I was confident enough I could cope. Still hopeful of stumbling on a house, I was averse to signing on anywhere I would have to work a month's notice. Once we had a home I wanted the children back immediately.

That left private nursing. I registered with an Agency and within days had a position that looked like salvation. Nine hours a day, at a stretch. No meal breaks. Three flights of stairs to the kitchen, two the toilet. Four pounds a day.

It was in my mind then, to work day and night if possible, seven days a week. I had to accumulate capital. Every evening after six, I'd walk to the Home to see the children, bathing the yougest and putting him to bed. He still clung and made the parting a pain. Then I'd walk back to wherever I was sleeping that night, the guest of kind friends, weighed down by weariness and the cross of separation.

From a large private house I moved to a small bed-sitter, sharing with a young teacher. She had the bed, I had the sitter. It was a long way from my work, and the Home. The bus drivers were on a go-slow strike. It meant taxis to my job. Fourteen hours on my feet and I couldn't get a bus back. This made such inroads into my salary I lay awake at night, fatigued as I was, doing sums in my fuddled mind. It wasn't working. As fast as I earned money it was running away as through a sieve, on tax, insurance and the price of living. My clothes needed replacing. Summer was coming. If I stayed on in the room where I was, I'd have the full rent to pay. Teachers have long holidays.

So do children. If they missed me in term time, as was evident, how much more so when they were not at school? It was bad enough now at weekends.

I began to take sedatives back with me from work, in a vain attempt to baffle my brain. All that did was give me nightmares and send me staggering to work with a head like an arthritic knee.

The strain was beginning to tell, and I could not work at the rate I intended. I had to have a day off. Then two. My health was failing. To save money I wasn't eating outside working hours.

Then one day I had an urgent call from the Sister in charge of Martin. Could I go down right away? He was ill and had a pain in his leg.

It shuddered through me. I had not kept my promise to him. Some nights I had satisfied conscience by just bathing the little one and not going on to see the others. He was in another house now, near the gate. It saved me the long, lone pilgrimage up the drive, and my precious time.

Full or remorse, I went to Martin now, and found a shy, thin child, delighted to see me but despising the fuss. He was in bed in the dormitory, and bored.

'He isn't eating and he can't walk,' Sister said anxiously.

'I'm not hungry,' he said cheerfully.

I knew the futility of trying to force appetite and reassured Sister it was not her fault. 'He's often like this. It goes off in a few days. I'll get him to a doctor when he can walk again.'

When we were alone he confessed he was happy at school, but he couldn't manage the walk there and back. He couldn't keep up with the others and was afraid of being late. The bus 'go-slow' was hitting him too. The Sisters were saving for a minibus, but in the meantime had no transport.

I made an appointment with the doctor who attended the Home, but when the day came I was unable to go. His sister took Martin, with a letter from me recording his history and symptoms. They called in on the way back to give me the verdict. 'He has probably pulled a muscle playing football. Rest it and bring him back in three weeks if he isn't any better.

Meantime the Home, in entirety, was going away to the coast. Martin loved the sand and sea. I persuaded him that since I was working anyway, he might just as well join them. He agreed, I was relieved to see some return of his mischief and pucking humour. Off school, he had picked up tremendously.

Just before they went, I found a flat I could rent furnished for the summer. It was upstairs; three small rooms and a kitchenette; no hot water without coal fire, outside toilet downstairs in the yard. Primitive by modern standards but paradise to me. I'd forgotten what it was like to sleep in a bed.

I moved in only just in time to stop my own constitution from disintegrating.

CHAPTER 5

Together again

During the next fortnight I began to understand why the priest had made that agreement. Motherhood, the way I had it, was a twice-round-the-clock job, every day of the year. No money of my own, no time to myself, never a day free of responsibility.

Now, for the first time in seventeen years I was on my own. The liberation was unbelievable.

The children completely safe and off my mind, except for daily correspondence, I was able to concentrate on myself. Shopping at leisure. Working out what I had been lacking in nutrition. Putting it right. Doing a bit of writing. Whole days off were such a novelty, I developed a new personality and shed years in a week.

With time to think, I began to realise there were organisations founded to help the homeless. At the rate I was going, I'd never re-house us myself. At the same time, my secure job, unlikely ever to be hit by redundancy, meant I could pay a mortgage.

I wrote off to a councillor I knew who had a SHELTER Group, and to the Catholic Building Society, which I also knew was sympathetic toward families. I had a long, confidential talk with a prominent member of the St Vincent de Paul Society.

Three estate agents had me on their lists and sent me details, at intervals, of property to view. A house came up that was just what we wanted; in a terrace, on a quiet road, near to schools, shops and churches. The Secretary of the Building Society promised to come up from London and have a look at it.

Martin came back, as cheeky and chirpy as his letters, to go straight on to Bristol with his sister. A friend of my late father's, knowing our sad situation, had offered them a week with him, and sent the fares. I waved them off, in the care of the guard. They were grown up and jumpy with excitement.

The five-year-old went with his brother down to Doncaster, to a big warm-hearted family I knew but had never met. I saw them off in the family van. They were willing but restrained. Then I went back to the convent to see the little one.

Sister met me, anxious and agitated. Martin had been sick the whole two weeks, she told me. 'He sat on the beach and didn't play at all. He's done nothing and eaten like a bird.'

I recalled the awkward way he had walked as we went for the train; as though he had a cannon-ball in his middle and had to negotiate around it. A niggle of fear wormed its way into my intuition. I sagged within, but comforted Sister and assured her, as soon as he came back we'd get something done about it.

The holidays at the foster-home were not a success. The two boys in Doncaster were found one day with forlorn faces and cases packed, silently pleading to come home. Martin and his sister enjoyed Longleat Park, the beautiful village, and the making of new friends. But they, too, suffered homesickness. Since we had no home, it was not so much a locality they missed as an axis; something psychologically stable around which life revolves, giving security. I was abysmally grieved and ashamed over the seeming ingratitude and slight toward the kind adults who took them, but with unselfish hearts that know children, they readily understood. After so much upheaval in their little lives, those youngsters must have wondered if they had been packed off away from me for ever.

Scarcely had they returned to the Home than the nuns asked if I'd taken them all out again. It was the convent annual rest period and they naturally wanted as many children as possible off the premises.

I had nowhere to take them but the flat, which was pitifully inadequate and not my property. I'd have to take the time away form work, which meant no money coming in, and keep us all, which meant money draining away.

On the other hand, there would be the luxury of getting to know them again, having them to myself, and not having to put them after a patient.

I agreed.

Change gave me the chance to take a good look at Martin, and confirm all Sister's anxiety. He was not eating; only odd platefuls of egg-and-bread fried. Nothing near what he needed to maintain health, growth and resistance. It occurred to me then why the cuffs of his coat were so long. He wasn't growing.

I went out that first day, stacked up with vitamins, food supplements, extra milk and anything nourishing he had ever fancied on the table.

His end-of-term report, despite his absences, showed him second top of his new class and had 'good' in five places. Martin was a good, hard-working boy. But Martin was not going to be able to stay that way unless something was done about his physical disability. I determined to get him to a doctor, near where we were, as soon as I could.

Meantime it was as much as I could do to feed the brood, protect the accommodation and cope with the mess. Overcrowding is bad for the nerves, and I felt the strain. Still, it was better than being separated.

Martin slept in a big, double bed with me, and I noticed that when we touched in his sleep, he winced, and moaned. Not only his leg but his spine seemed tender. I put a soft pillow between us.

He never complained. I could get nothing out of him about the past three months, but, 'Oh, it was all right.' It was his sister who told me he often cried at nights. Sometimes he'd sit by the window alone, waiting for me to come, till time was gone and hope had died. It couldn't have been. But it must have seemed eternity to him.

I blazed in my mind at the cruelty of a world that could inflict such deep unhappiness on so young a child. I vowed there and then he would never leave me again. If I had to take him to work with me, we were staying together.

That summer I'd recorded a television Epilogue all about Martin. He had such a shrewd line in reasoning, his bland proof of the existence of God had amazed me, and I used the incident. We were all at the flat when the programme was transmitted and stayed up till midnight to watch.

Martin was lost in delirious enjoyment, but wordless till the end. Then he turned to me with eyes all sparks and said 'That was great!' It was for him the absolute ultimate in appreciation, and gave me a sublime thrill. I promised I'd use him again, whenever the was struck by genius.

I had also made an appointment with the doctor and, the night before, decided to strip Martin and wash him. He was a shy, self-reliant child, much more independent now since the Home. There was no hot water at the flat but what we could boil in a kettle so washing was a slap-happy, only-the-bits-that show affair. They were on holiday, I was relaxing, I wasn't too hard on them.

But this night I got the others away to bed, to get Martin fit for inspection. He protested it wasn't necessary; doctors didn't expect boys to be clean, but I insisted. He obeyed. He was still ticklish and giggling, but enjoyed the renewal of an old relationship.

I slipped off his vest. My eyes took in the spare shoulders, and thin arms, then slipped down and riveted to his waist. My hands dropped as though slapped and I leaned back on my heel aghast. From under his skinny rib-cage came a swelling out of all proportion to his size.

A chill hit my brain. It was abnormal.

'Come on,' he urged, impatient, 'I'm goose-pimpling. Get on with it!'

I rallied and finished him gently, ideas slipping through my nurse's mind like well-oiled chain. Swelling. Pain. Weight loss. No appetite. Anaemia. No energy. Relentless syndrome; recurring, progressive getting worse. Oh my God.

Sublimating knowledge I smacked his

bottom, saw to his teeth and put him into bed. We said our prayers as ever, together, and added, 'Please God make Martin eat.' He giggled again, rarely serious these days, and settled down ecstatically with his comics. To be lying there, that late at night, with me pottering about the flat where he could hear, was his interpretation of Heaven.

I hummed as I worked, but under it I panicked. Where had I seen that shape of his before; that ungainly, unnatural potential taken to extreme? Training, Ward days? No, they were too remote.

Biafra! That was it. The papers were full of it. Biafran babies dying of malnutrition. Pathetically distended centrally, surrounded by bones.

But Martin had been so well cared for, so lovingly supervised. He was eating something. He wasn't starving. How could he be like them? *Where* was all the nourishment going?

I had to get him a taxi to the surgery; double fare because it came from town. It was a large, modern group practice.

The doctor was friendly and ready. He made Martin wait outside while I told the story. He sensed my distress.

When Martin came in, he jovially got him relaxed and responsive, then gave him a thorough examination. I sat, counting beads in my head, knowing so much but not enough; dependent on this man's experience.

'Well,' he said at last, as Martin slipped eagerly off the couch and back to me, 'There doesn't seem anything there to worry about.'

I was disappointed and it showed.

'The swelling isn't all that bad,' he expanded.

I felt an absolute fool.

'As for the eating. I shouldn't let it upset you,' lightly. 'One of a large family. Probably trying to get attention.' He laughed. 'I have one myself just like him. Goes on hunger strike when he thinks he's being ignored.'

He was being reassuring but I didn't want that. I wanted truth. Injustice flared in me. Martin had never needed to bid for attention. As for striking, he wasn't the type.

I told the doctor what I was giving him, perhaps to show that I was trying.

He laughed out loud. 'Vitamins? A chemist's racket! Just a fad. He gets all he needs from a normal balanced diet.'

I started to say, 'But he isn't *eating* a normal, balanced diet...' The words died unsaid. I was beginning to sound like a crank.

There *was* very little to see, now we were in the surgery. He had ruled out several major disorders that were written on my mind. That was something to be thankful for.

We made for the door.

'Bring him back in a week or two if you're not satisfied. We'll take it from there.'

I nodded. I wasn't satisfied. But the owner of the flat was coming back and we had nowhere to go. God alone knew where we would be 'in a week or two.'

CHAPTER 6

The truth

The Secretary of the Building Society, true to his word, came north and investigated our case. He met the children, saw the way we were living, viewed the house, realised the urgency and went back promising to do what he could.

Shortly after that I had promising news about a grant towards the deposit. We were all anticipation.

The children wound up their school holidays with a visit to the television studios to watch me doing a recording. They were in turn excited, awed, impressed and utterly unmoved. Rarely did they react as expected. The floor manager made their day by presenting them each with a giant ball-point pen; a bigger thrill by far than seeing their mother on television.

Martin was deeply, wonderfully interested and pleaded to be taken again.

When the time came for the return to the Home, the youngest made a terrible scene. Having had a taste of family life again, he knew what he was missing. The institution and everybody in it was alien. My heart went out to the Sister who had come to love him as I did. She was his mother too. But she was leaving. I had to decide whether to leave him or take him and I chose the latter. His security was in jeopardy.

Regretfully I sent a letter of resignation to my employer, explaining the circumstances. I was no longer a working mother.

On September the 4th I took the two boys on a day trip to York, to the home of St Margaret Clitherow, one of the English Martyrs. It was a pilgrimage, for a home, and Martin. His dragging leg made it difficult, but he said it wasn't meant to be easy; it was a penance.

A few days later a generous girl from

the studios offered us a room at her house until the purchase of ours was completed. We packed our trunk, said goodbye to the flat, and the three of us like nomads moved on.

It was comfort and rest and a breathing space, but it was not destined to last. The other children wanted to come. When they came they wanted to stay. Martin's leg was getting worse. The husband of the house told me about an osteopath he knew who had worked miracles of manipulation and healing. I determined to take Martin. Anxiety had given way to conviction. This could not be ignored.

That Sunday we had a birthday party for one of the boys. Martin's brother brought me a re-addressed letter. It was to inform me that our application for a grant towards the deposit on the house had been turned down. We were refugees.

In desperation I telephoned another nun I knew; the headmistress of an approved school for girls, run by the Order of the Good Shepherd. She had once before offered me a room for myself. I told her what had happened and asked if she could possibly put up the boys too.

'Just bring them,' she said. 'We'll think about that when you get here.'

With all the relief of Mary and Joseph shown the stable on Christmas Eve, we jumped at the offer.

We fell on feathers.

Sister gave us the sick bay, which was empty and due for structural alteration. There was a bedroom, bathroom and use of a kitchen. Some meals we could obtain from the school dining-room, others we could prepare ourselves. We were free to come and go as we pleased, and enjoy the grounds.

We made one journey more, back to the previous address, to collect what we had left. The couple were away. Two of the other children had previously arranged to meet us there and weren't to know we had gone. They were irritated and truculent at yet another change, but I cheered them with an optimistic vision and said (like the shepherds) 'Come and see.'

Laden, we took the trail back to the station.

It was warm. The trains ran infrequently. Ours was standing at the platform over the bridge as I bought the tickets.

'Run!' I told the two who were fleetest, 'Go tell the guard we're on our way. He'll wait.' Struggling with a child and two cases, I passed Martin, who couldn't hurry, and assured him I'd be back for him.

As I descended the steps at the other side, to my horror, the guard blew his whistle and signalled the train to leave. Pop-eyed, through the window of a closed carriage, two anguished faces told me a tale. He hadn't listened to their appeal and had bundled the pair of them in.

'Stop!' I yelled. 'Please...There's another...' and leaving the little one as hostage, I streaked back to get Martin.

I couldn't hurry either, by then. Panting, I climbed the stairs, crossed the bridge and looked down.

Never, to my last day, will I be able to forget what met me.

Martin, convinced he was being left behind, had been getting up as best he could, in a panic and a frenzy only the disabled can know. He'd heard the whistle and had fallen in a spasm; clutching, crawling, weeping, mauling his own body to move, he was in agony. And close by, fully aware of his struggle, two porters were idly talking.

They had seen what was going on. They knew very well we were after that train. They could see the child was handicapped. They just didn't care.

At that point, to the redemption of my faith in men, another official dashed out of the office. He'd seen it too. In one move he picked Martin off the steps, got him safe in his arms, and carried him bodily over the bridge. He made the guard wait, giving me time to reach them, then bundled us all in. I didn't even have time to thank him.

The train moved. The children cried.

Quietly Martin clung to me in mortification. His spine was rigid, his legs in a tremor, I shared each shuddering breath, my coat wet with his frustrated tears.

Strangers stared. One passenger was plainly irritated. Not a soul moved toward our group in compassion, let alone sympathy. It was our first experience of the callous inhumanity of the public towards the handicapped.

It was not to be our last.

The girls at the school, though, made up for it in an hour. Failures they may have been, in sight of law and society, but to us they were Salvation. Hospitable and uninhibited, they recognised no convention, knew no restraint. They took us in as an R.S.P.C.A. voluntary worker takes sick animals from the street.

For Martin, especially, they had a rough and ready love that was healing in itself. Separated from home and family themselves, betrayed by life, they seemed to see in us all that was unhappiness. And wanted to help. They took the children along to their family groups, fed them, spoiled them, played with them. Children are sensitive to atmosphere and they opened up like sunflowers. When I was alone, the girls came to me with their crimes and confessions. They made me feel important. I was amazed at how innocent, under God, so many of them were. Just trapped by circumstances; born into a bad world. It was noisy and tiring when I needed peace, but it gave me a sound basis to fall back on when the next blow came.

During the night after we arrived, I saw Martin climb quietly out of bed. His back was curved, as though about to snap. His shoulders were hunched. He leaned on the bed as a walking stick, and walked like a little old man.

I made no sign, but waited until he was back and asleep. Then stunned by dark premonition, I turned and wept till I slept.

Next day we all went to Mass in the convent chapel. Martin had missed sometimes because he couldn't sit upright. His spine would not support him for long. Today, however, he wanted to go, to be among the girls. I prayed for patience, faith and ability to accept whatever came. I tried to trust the Good Shepherd, as these Sisters did.

Half way through the Gospel, Martin sat up, grabbed the rail, slipped sideways and fell, with a thud, in a heap at my feet. His spine had completely given way.

One of the staff bent instantly to pick him up, and carried him out. I stayed behind, to calm the others and avoid a scene. He was not unconscious and he trusted her. But I boiled within that all this could be brushed aside as normal and of no significance.

After Mass, with Martin resting, I told Sister all my thoughts. She suggested I take him to the casualty department of the city infirmary the very next day.

The gardener took us in, by minibus. He lifted Martin out limp as a baby, found a wheelchair and gently laid him down. I went across to the desk, and the receptionist, 'This child cannot walk,' I told her, as steadily as I was able. 'Will somebody please find out why.'

The doctor on duty was clearly uncertain, so sent for the children's registrar. He came down, listened to the history, then carefully examined Martin.

The child was obviously terrified. It was his first experience of hospital since an accident with a swing when he was a toddler. They'd taken him away, screaming that day, to have his brow stitched, and left me outside. This time I hovered near, where he could see me. He was unnatural, apprehensive and restrained, but he co-operated. The doctor smiled at him and came over to me.

'The trouble is in his hip I think. Impossible to tell from here.' He glanced apologetically at Martin. 'We'll have to have him in I'm afraid.'

Martin began to cry, his face puckered in dismay. 'Oh no,' he whined. 'I'm not staying in here. I won't, I won't, I won't.' I felt for him. Another separation. Something else to dread.

It took a while but I did manage to convince him this was necessary and for the best. Once he realised it had my full consent, and that I could come in any time, he accepted it, I saw him in to the ward and into bed. Then I went out and bought him what he had been promised for his birthday, two weeks ahead. He was going to be alone again and insecure. He needed it now.

The girls were livid at his detention and protested even louder than he did. 'He doesn't need to stay in hospital! We can look after him.' They all went back to their flats and wrote him long letters of heated emotion.

I wrote to him too; long typed letters giving him faith and hope and love; dealing methodically with all I knew he feared, and his native pessimism.

Tests were under way; all of them strange, some painful. Every time I went, he greeted me with tears. He would not attempt to integrate into the ward routine and lay pining until I came. The registrar, knowing well what was listed in my mind, relieved me as each disease was discarded.

On the third day, the consultant asked if he could see me alone. We had just had a jovial exchange around Martin's bed. I was unprepared for gravity.

The registrar came along, and they took me into the office. They sat me down and clicked on a light under a chest X-ray. There were what seemed like bits of fluff on the rib-cage. I wanted to dust them off.

'These are metasteses.' The consultant said. 'Whatever the initial condition, I'm afraid it's malignant.'

There was no impact. It was as though my mind had been cushioned. My reaction was of interest rather than shock. How could I be shocked? Hadn't I known for weeks what the verdict would be?

'There's liver involvement,' he went on kindly. 'We'll know how much after the biopsy.'

Liver biopsy. I shrank from it. Painful, and slow healing. Such a deep operation, to prove...what?

He asked our circumstances and I told him briefly.

'You've had it rough,' he said.

I shrugged. 'It's life.'

I thanked them and went back into the ward, as though I'd just been to make a telephone call.

That night I slept in Martin's bed and bit hard into the pillow, trying to believe it, a deep tormenting grief ripping my soul. Martin had cancer. My Martin. My baby. My little boy.

Martin had cancer. Cancer. CANCER! My angel, my comforter, eaten away inside, by a crab. All this time and nobody heeded me. Nobody listened to me. Nobody believed.

I thought of all the terminals I had nursed; They slipped through my head like coloured slides. Morphia. Mutilation. Sallow, yellow skins. Surgery. Radium. Sickness. Death. Slow. Quick. No other end. Inevitable.

Next morning early I went into the chapel and prayed. 'Please God, make it easy for Martin. Make it easy for him.' There was no doubt in my mind but that he would die. The registrar said 'two months,' if we hadn't brought him in, but what difference would it make?

I took it, as I take everything in life, as the will of God for me. It knows no why. We're all born to die.

I waited until I had the courage to face the world, and then I told Sister.

I didn't want it getting around. I couldn't cope with enquiries. But I found it worse, when anybody asked anxiously 'How's Martin?', if I tried to lie. I told them we weren't very sure what it was, but it was incurable.

The girls, as a group, fell to mourning and weeping. *They* were shocked. They had me bringing get-well cards and gifts for them to send to him.

'Don't worry Miss,' one red-headed rebel said, 'We'll look after him. We'll get him better for yer. They don't know nothin' in them places. They don't know nothin'.'

They knew a lot more when I went again. Martin had a neuroblastoma; tumour of the gland attached to his kidney. There were secondaries in the liver, and they didn't need a biopsy; an X-ray was sufficient.

Thankful for that, I enquired about his hip. It was fibrositis; pressure and fluid. No disease there. I stifled a 'not yet' in myself, and went in to see Martin.

'Good news,' I told him playfully. 'You can smile again. They're not going to do any more tests. You're coming out.'

CHAPTER 7

Happy Birthday

While Martin was still in the Infirmary I met an acquaintance who dealt in property. He had just purchased a large, derelict house to convert into flats and, hearing our plight, said we could use the middle floor meantime, for up to a month or two.

It was damp, dark and dirty, full of fusty furniture, sour beer bottles and mice. But it did have possibilities and was better than despair. We couldn't stay where we were indefinitely.

Martin didn't like the house. He had a sensitive nature and an eye for beauty, plus his dependence on physical ease. He came once, decided he couldn't stand the smell and from then on stayed away. The girls, however, who were used to scrubbing a cathedral, fell on it like excited marauders. A home? They'd soon have it habitable; They packed into the minibus and descended on the house with buckets, cloths, detergent, abrasive powders, disinfectant and traps for the mice. It worked some of the revolt out of them and gave them a sense of achievement.

Meanwhile Martin had started his treatment, as an outpatient. Two drugs, vincristine and cyclophosphamide, had had some success in other cases. It was hoped they would inhibit the tumour growth. I was warned that they might have some side-effects, anaemia, bleeding from the bladder and his hair falling out, but the risks seemed worth taking, to prolong his life. I had been asked by the research unit for a blood sample myself, and it was found to contain antibodies, so the condition was congenital. It was also, obviously, slow-growing.

I started a case-book on the day he was diagnosed. From now on he was going to be my private patient, and have all the benefit of what I had learned on others.

I began to read everything I could find on malignancy, including books by so-called 'cranks'. One thing struck me forcibly. The growths were but symptoms of a systemic condition. Strengthen the entire system, and we could probably fight the disease.

Here I hit a dilemma. Quite obviously, if I nourished the child I was also nourishing the tumour. Was that a wise thing to do? Yet what was the alternative; to starve them both? There are nutritional elements essential for the proper working of a human body. What would his life be without energy, vitality and resistance to other ailments ever threatening a child? I settled for feeding the child, sensibly and reasonably and left the tumour to look after itself.

The effect of the drugs on Martin's system, however, held up any plans involving good. It was disastrous, and nothing like what I had been warned. He had diarrhoea, he vomited incessantly, ate nothing at all wasn't even able to drink. So much for my strengthening campaign.

His interest in people was gone completely. He just lay in bed, looking blue and ashen, alternately dozing and moaning, for hours on end. Three days after the injection, these effects began to wear off. By the fifth, he was beginning to be himself again. On the seventh he was due another injection.

So I sat up one night, by his bed, torturing myself through to another decision. Drugs I had never had much use for, especially in their experimental stages. I had nursed too many unpleasant side-effects. This treatment was becoming worse than the disease, and ruining what little life he had left. The simple pleasure he had was being wrested from him. The quality of life was more, far more, than its length. I had accepted that he had not very long to live. So long as he was going to die, he would die happy. I wrote to the registrar telling him exactly how I felt, and asked for the drugs to be stopped. In reply I was given an appointment with the child surgeon now in charge of Martin's case.

He was not pessimistic about the situation and explained that the drug dosage had been drastic to start with; almost certain to be a shock to the system. The child was being given a crash course, in an attempt to arrest the tumour. As the dose was decreased, he felt sure, the sickness would disappear. So I let it ride for a while. The specialist also mentioned that there has been occasional instances of spontaneous disappearance of such a tumour. I was grateful for his trying to give me hope, but I knew, and so did he, that secondaries of liver and chest don't also spontaneously disappear. That takes a miracle.

In view of my financial straits, I was referred to the Malcolm Sargent relief fund, which paid us a small weekly allowance. There was also a voluntary fund at the Children's Clinic which would pay him to have a taxi to his monthly appointment, when he was weighed and examined. The injections he had weekly, on the ward.

From then on, for about two days a

week he ate normally, slept normally, was interested in life and able to get about. The other five he was felled by the drugs and life came to a complete stop. Then the drugs were separated, given alternate weeks, and it became apparent it was the cyclophosphamide that upset him. He came to dread it, and to plead not to go. I had to be stern, but my sympathy was all with him. Was it not enough to be handicapped and disabled, unable to do as others did, without this addition of digestive illness and stupor?

October 17th was his 10th birthday. An air of hushed excitement swirled about in the Grange. Martin contained his anticipation, but he knew very well what was under way. The girls had planned a surprise party, in one of the 'families'. It was their own idea, and their own money.

By this time, his brother and sister, still in care of the Sisters of Nazareth, were frequent visitors, and it was becoming harder each time they came, to get them to go back. I told our Sister at the Grange, who responded immediately.

'Let them stay.' She had seen the effects of mother deprivation and felt their need of me. The older children, still living at other addresses till we had a home, had been secretly invited to the party, so on Martin's big day, for the first time in five months, seven children would be together again.

The party flat, when we were all ushered in, was breath-taking. No wonder they had kept us all out of the way. The tables were laden to every possible taste. Balloons and streamers obscured the ceiling and walls. There were comic hats, loads of novelties, and centre of it all, a cake that would send any ten-year-old pop-eyed. One of the staff had fashioned and iced it as a genuine football field, with players in Martin's local colours. It was incredibly real, and merited being painted in oils.

Martin was just getting over an injection, so couldn't eat a lot, but feasted his eyes and his soul. He overcame his nausea to join in all the games, and enjoyed everything that came his way. Letters and cards kept being delivered, from all the places he had recently been. Everyone, it seemed, was determined to make it a birthday to remember, and underlying all, with a tug that would not be denied, was the fact that it may well be his last.

Just to make everything right, we had just heard that in view of our heavy disappointment over the housing grant, the building society had decided to raise its loan. We could buy the house we wanted after all.

'Thank goodness,' Martin said flatly. 'Now we don't need that dingy one.'

It was a drained, exhausted boy I rolled into bed that night, long after the young ones were asleep. 'Wasn't it great?' he said wearily, his face lit from inside with soft light and memories.

'Great,' I repeated.

Too tired for words he said his prayers in his head, and drifted off I thought. I was arranging his cards on the dressing table, busying myself near him as ever, when a peaceful little voice came to me out of the darkness. 'Mam' it said clearly.

'This has been the happiest day of my life.'

I nodded and smiled, and trusted to the dark to hide my tears. It had indeed. Thank God for the nuns. Thank God for the delinquents. Thank God for the Good Shepherd. He couldn't have timed it better.

CHAPTER 8

A new relationship

Just before we moved, it was decided that something must be done about Martin's anaemia. It was making him weak and breathless, and could be rectified easily by blood transfusion. The big problem was, telling Martin he had to go into hospital again.

I knew exactly how he would feel. His introduction to that environment had been harsh, radical and painful. He was always glad to get away after his injection on the ward, his new confidence there being in the knowledge that he could. The disease itself affected his central nervous system, making him jumpy and unusually apprehensive. Few boys of his age are brave about physical pain anyway, and this new experience could only alarm him unduly. It was also going to test his faith in me. I'd known of this possibility, but had kept it from him, so as not to have its shadow over everything we did. He had to feel free, while he *was* free, and not have anything to spoil it.

But I saw a road ahead that was going to involve many a difficult corner such as this. I had to work out a way of handling it. I didn't want him to go. Every minute away from him, now, I felt I was losing a slipping rein. He was precious as he had never been, and God knows he was dear enough before. To be detached and unemotional in such circumstances, taking the entire responsibility for breaking bad news, and then getting obedience was not easy.

'Martin,' I said, taking him aside from the rest for a talk on the settee one afternoon. 'I have two things to tell you. One bad, one good.'

His face fell. He had an intuition about unpleasantness that robbed me of my advantage. I pressed on 'Which do you want first?'

'The bad,' he said gloomily. 'Get it over.'

'All right then,' I took a breath 'You have to go back into hospital.'

His face crumpled.

'It's only for a day or two,' I consoled.

'But we're moving,' he wailed.

'You'll come back into the new house. All ready for you.'

'Oh no'...he refused, and fell to punching the cushion hard. 'I'm not going back into that place, I'm not, I'm not, I'm NOT.'

'You've got to.'

Taking a hold of him I steadied him and told him straight. 'If you don't, you won't be any good, for anything. All the things I said we would do together. All the places I've promised you we'll go. You'll be so tired all the time I'll have to carry you, and you know how far we'll get that way.

'I know I promised you I wouldn't send you away again, but this is different. It's only another injection really. But it takes longer and you have to lie very still. They can't do it here.'

He was intelligent enough to reason, and he knew when I had made up my mind. He gave in and hid his face on me.

'I don't want it Martin,' I held him hard. 'But it has to be. Something we just have to face together.'

'You come with me mind,' he insisted, sitting up at last, 'and you sit by my bed the whole time.'

The selfishness of the dependent. I had the other children to see to, and a removal to organise.

'I can't promise, but somebody will be there, and I'll have you out as soon as it's over.'

'You didn't tell me the good thing.'

'Oh,' I brightened to brighten him. 'How would you like to go to Lourdes?'

His mouth fell open and his eyes lit.

'On an aeroplane,' I tempted. 'All the way to France.'

'Lourdes. Oh yes.' He thought, beamed and lightened. 'That would be great.'

'Don't tell anybody,' I warned. 'You'll only make them all want to go. But you see, you'll have to be fit, or the hospital won't let you go.'

We were round the corner. He accepted the worst, looking forward to the best, and passively if not cheerfully went through his ordeal. We took it in turns to sit with him, so he was never alone, except when he was asleep. The hospital staff were kindness itself and the operation was quite painless. He came out with fresh roses in his cheeks, and pink in the tips of his ears.

'When are we going to Lourdes?', was one of the first things he asked me when we were on our own.

I had no idea I was penniless and tied. I was just quite determined I would get him there, and there was a call in me. 'I'm not sure,' I countered easily. 'We have a few strings to pull. You pray, I'll start writing letters.'

He did more than that. The practical imp got an old red box once used for flag-selling, put a label on the front 'Lourdes Fund', and put it on the bar-top in the lounge. Visitors got the message and the offerings began to be quietly dropped in.

Meanwhile I had six children in the house, and no income but what the State saw fit to pay me. I couldn't do any outside work. My brain ever more maternal than mathematical, struggled endlessly with bills that always took me by surprise. We managed but we were dependent on charity and felt it.

I couldn't possibly do everything expected of me. I had to make a list of priorities. Routine, obviously, had to revolve around Martin and his needs. He did enjoy being with the other children, but noise affected him adversely, and I didn't want him snapping at them when they got on his nerves. He had to have a hide-away. That apart, the prognosis searing my mind, I knew the kindest way, for all the family, was to detach them from him, gently. I put him in a large attic on the top floor and I took the room next to it. I knew what could well develop, I had to be near, and I didn't want him perhaps upsetting or disturbing the others.

The stairs were a problem; two long flights, with curves. His leg trouble hadn't eased any, and exercise had to be carefully gauged, or he suffered pain. The doctor had assured me, however, that there was no disease in his hip—only fluid. It was a matter of strict regulation to avoid distress. We cut the excursions up and downstairs to an absolute minimum, and enlisted the big boys to carry him when they were in. I didn't want him paralysing their lives and movements or they would come to resent him, but there was usually somebody around when he wanted a lift.

His diet was still my main preoccupation, and no easy task. I knew what he ought to have; getting it into him was a tricky proposition. His appetite was fickle. For so long, his illness apparently a transitory thing, he had been allowed to eat just what he fancied. Now I had to wean him away from the fizzy drinks and fries, to get essential protein, vitamins, calcium, minerals and fruit in. He didn't like milk. He wasn't hungry when there was a meal prepared, and was when it wasn't. It was going to be important to prevent the toxins from building up in his system, making him *feel* ill as well as being so. Things like carrot juice have such a cleansing action, but what boy of his age would be excited by that proposition?

At last, frustrated and becoming angry at so much wasted effort on my part, I sat him down and explained the position. 'Look Martin. You don't eat because you like eating. You don't eat only what you like. You eat because food to you is like petrol to a car. Without it the engine won't go. Put water in, or coke, and your car is in trouble. We can't go anywhere. I don't give you anything that isn't exactly what your motor needs. If you want to be mobile, you've just got to get it into you, somehow.'

I was rarely annoyed with him. He knew when I meant business. He looked suitably abashed. 'I have a nasty taste all the time,' he confessed. 'And I feel full up.'

I fought back maternal sympathy. 'That's all right. It will go if you eat the right things. You're filling yourself up with thick things like buns and beans, so there's no room for the oranges and eggs. And the mixtures I make to wash them down. I'll still give you the things and tastes you like, but you must eat the diet first.'

He agreed, without much enthusiasm, but it soon became a fascinating game. We worked on the permutations of food values, did a tour of health food shops and herbalists, and found a dozen ways to get each essential into him. Variety and concentrates stimulated his appetite. Carrot, we found, combined well with apple juice. He didn't like it, but he mastered it, and made no complaint. Wheat germ he took in capsules, with no difficulty at all, cutting out the need for bread.

'The Diet' had become an institution, funny to everybody but us. Iron and liver, I hoped, would ward off the need for further transfusions, and prevent further separation. Experts on dietary requirements as far apart as Dublin and Edinburgh, took an interest in Martin's case. Each consignment of supplies was accompanied by a note enquiring about his progress and response. Amongst us, despite his illness and his recurring nausea, we provided a completely natural source of energy and protection, free of artificial colouring and preservatives, white flour and white sugar, all in a form he could assimilate and even enjoy.

The only kick-back was on me, ironically. Martin threw at me, with usual cheek one day. 'Hey, what about you? Don't you take vitamins? You have an engine too.'

He was so right. I had the strain of the entire household, his condition, and a fund of emotional stresses enough to bring any chassis to a halt. From then on I watched my own diet, and never regretted it. I have a great deal to thank him for. Without a fortified constitution, the life I had, I'd have succumbed to a complete breakdown in a very short time.

His sickness persisted, especially after

the cyclophosphamide, and was a recurring set-back that upset us both. He was otherwise improving in so many ways. Seeing the drug dragging him, I tried again to get it stopped. The specialist was reluctant to drop his only medical hope, and we argued for a bit. I was so much more concerned that Martin was not *made* to feel ill, by a foreign cause, and that nature could have complete freedom to do her own work.

He still couldn't walk far without his leg giving way. This was noticed, and I let it be known that he was handicapped. There was no earthly point in distressing kind people with the truth. The unkind didn't care anyway. There was no necessity to warn Martin that he may not have long to live. It could do nothing but shake his security. His greatest fear, and his biggest effort, when it became necessary, was separation from me. What nightmare could there be for him in the knowledge that we would have to part indefinitely? I was so preoccupied anyway with the joy of keeping him comfortable and happy, attending to his needs, I completely forgot what was wrong with him, till something or somebody reminded me. We lived for the present, took what came, and made the most of it, spending as much time as we possibly could together.

I had explained to him that we had something inside him, like a ball, that was causing the swelling. The doctors couldn't take it out without hurting everything else, but it was nothing to worry about. It accounted for the swelling and his difficulty in manipulating into a sitting position. Discomfort was his constant companion, but he alleviated it in his own curious ways. He liked best to curl up flat on the floor, like a cat, and had a similar attraction to the fire.

I was afraid of my lonely, sole responsibility. Every time a new symptom seemed to appear, such as a nose-bleed, I had a wave of panic. Was it secondaries? He was so trusting, and so utterly flexible under my reasoning. Was I doing the right thing? It was, strangely, his own utter ignorance of the truth that strengthened me. He was so active, within his limitations, so intelligent, such good company, and so obviously alive.

From the very beginning I turned him to God and the Faith he knew. I was possessed of my own helplessness and needed somewhere to send him. I never forced him to anything, but encouraged him to go to Mass, and to Communion. Calling in at church was as natural as going to the shops. He knew that feeding up his body was only a part of living. His spirit needed nourishing too.

Just once he cornered me, as I was working in his room. 'Mam', he said practically, not troubling to look up from his game. 'If the doctors can't find a cure for me, what are we going to do?'

'Go to God,' I answered him naturally, easily. 'Whatever they can't do, God can.'

It was enough. The moment passed. Another corner rounded. Whether God really would or not was another matter; a question for tomorrow. We lived for the moment. It was enough to know, God *could* do the impossible.

CHAPTER 9

Happy Christmas

By December, Martin's condition seemed to be resolving. The drugs had been reduced, and his sickness was not so frequent or so obvious. He was eating better. He still took a long time to pull round in the mornings, but once up, he was downstairs most of the day. He wasn't gaining weight, but nor was he losing any, which seemed to suggest he was holding his own.

Bad weather considerably cut down his outings. The bus strike was still on. Times we did decide to make a break for it, to relieve the monotony, it was a case of waiting around bus shelters till Martin was too weak to stand. Then he'd curl up in his relaxed heap on the ground, attracting disparaging glances from passers-by.

We didn't do that very often.

I was still doing a little television though, and occasionally was asked to speak at a meeting. Anywhere I had transport provided I took Martin with me. Not only was he fascinated by anything and everything I did, his lively mind stimulated mine, all too often suffering from fatigue.

Lourdes was becoming a definite project, with various ideas and plans taking shape. I had the promise from a young teacher friend that she would come and supervise the other children, to let me take Martin away for a week-end. To crown her offer, we were given the opportunity of two free places on a weekend pilgrimage in February. The Society of St Vincent de Paul, hearing the news, provided my fare to London. A wonderful priest who had met Martin only once, insisted on paying the rest. Our financial position, generally, was extremely insecure, but this was marked money and I refused to touch it for any other purpose.

Unfortunately, I had also run into

trouble with the law. Considerably under the weather one dreadful morning, I made a stupid mistake in a supermarket, and was spotted by a store detective. Unable to see the difference between confusion and criminal intent, she had me arrested for shoplifting. My good name *sub judice* as it were, I had to drop all my public work and fight to clear it. Tension and uncertainty hung over me for three months, but Martin was unaware of it.

Just before Christmas, the specialist expressed the opinion that Martin was fit enough to go to school. I wasn't sure. I knew his low capacity for physical strain. We had no transport, and the nearest school was half a mile away. I couldn't pay for taxis every day. His brilliant mind did need developing though, and I didn't want him to miss schooling. I saw the headmistress, and explained the position. She agreed that he would be relieved of anything but absolute essentials.

Martin looked on it with mixed feelings, as will any boy seeing the end of an extended holiday. He didn't protest, or even question the arrangement, but I could see he was dreading the undertaking. 'What happens if I get a pain?' he asked me.

'You come home,' I said firmly, 'and you don't go back until it's absolutely all gone.'

He sighed, inside. His consciousness of his weaknesses was something that persistently evaded other people, but never me. I felt it as though it were my own. I did try, once, to get him into a group for handicapped children, thinking there would be normality in the grading down of effort required. It was a club night when we went, and Martin lasted about twenty minutes. He couldn't stand the noise, and he was shaken to his soul by the sight of mentally retarded among the physically handicapped.

'Oh Mam,' he said, unhappily, pulling my sleeve. 'I'm not nearly as bad as them. Let's go home.'

I had to apologise afterwards to the good people who ran the club. But it was intended to help, and that wasn't what

Martin needed. He was far better in his own home surroundings, with his own family, doing just as he felt able to, as and when he pleased. I never tried to get him to join anything again.

For Christmas, we relied entirely on Providence. Poverty was our lot, and there was little we could give, even to each other. Word had got around, though, and things began to arrive, especially for Martin. I had to explain to him that it wasn't fair if I gave everything to him. The others were going to feel terribly left out, and he had two brothers younger than himself. Without a murmur, he agreed to share. He even told me what I should give them. The only things he was possessive about were those that stimulated his mind, and which he relied upon for activity when the others went out to play. These he guarded carefully, knowing what juvenile borrowing and carelessness can do. I never asked him to share them. I guarded them as he did.

We trusted to God, but he cannot provide without people who will give, and they did Him justice over the holidays. Food hampers, letters of hope and help, remembrance from people we felt sure must have forgotten by then. An ex-alcoholic we had never met sent Martin a toy tank he had made himself. Somehow there was enough to go round.

On January 5th Martin started school. We had permission for him to wear long trousers; his legs were so pathetically thin. With a flat piece across the front, and waist elasticated, they made the swelling around his middle scarcely noticable. He still hadn't grown into his coat. He looked so cheerful, and so vulnerable, it made me choke to leave him, but he wanted to go. A boy for the boys, he wanted to be part of life, and live as they did. I wasn't really bothered about his making friends. It was the walking that troubled me. He had to come home for lunch; the school couldn't possibly cope with what he ate. It was a long trek, four ways each day, and he tired easily.

We solved this, a little later; he borrowed his sister's bicycle. It was much too high, and difficult for him to manipulate as well as control, but he managed, and it did take the weight from his legs. He was the only boy in the school with permission to take a bicycle, which sent him up in the eyes of his mates.

One day, he came in very tearful, declaring outrage at the educational establishment. Sister, the headmistress, had allowed him to stay in the classroom at play-times, in case the boys got boisterous and did him accidental damage. Rough play did unnerve him; he was unsteady on his feet and hadn't much stamina. He also felt the cold keenly. He was quite happy to sit by the radiator and read. That day, though, the caretaker had come in, thought he was lagging behind, and ordered him out with the others. He was angry and truculent.

I didn't like to see him rebellious. It was a trait he was rapidly losing. He had to realise that life was going to be hard, and not be soft under it. He mustn't misjudge other people, no matter how they misjudged him. There was virtue developing in this child; real manliness. I didn't want him thrown back into baby immaturity by what was obviously misunderstanding.

'It's your own fault,' I said lightly, not moving from what I was doing. 'You look so darned healthy, and you seem just like the others. How did you expect her to know the difference?'

It pleased him. He stopped, and thought, and forgave her immediately. Then he forgot. He wasn't one for holding a grudge.

On January 7th, my birthday, there was a school test, to grade the boys into places. Martin came home with a beaming grin, and a cheeky nonchalance. 'I'm top of the class,' he said. It quieted something questing in me. It seemed to normalise everything.

Next day he was off school to go to the clinic for his monthly check up. Coming back from the X-ray department, I had a look at the result. I couldn't believe it. His chest X-ray was clear. No secondaries. I waited till we had seen the specialist, and confirmed it, before I told Martin.

'Yippee,' he said, over his coke, which we always had to wind up a session at the Infirmary. He was walking so well, within his limits, that we did the homeward journey under our own steam.

'More than that,' I congratulated, 'It's three months since you had that blood transfusion, and you don't need another one.' It was certainly full marks for the team.

He sucked slowly for a few seconds, then said quietly, with a calm sagacity. 'Of course you know why that is. I've got the best private nurse.'

It got me right behind the eyes. Gratitude is so rare in a child. He seemed to be growing up in leaps and jumps.

We needed that boost though. The court case was dragging on over my shoplifting. It was going to have to go to quarter sessions. We couldn't possibly leave the country, not even to take a dying child to Lourdes. All over a jar of malted milk costing less than 40p, we had to cancel the pilgrimage, and of course, we lost the free places. Martin was disappointed, but not unduly perturbed. It was a little cold for travelling, in February. 'We'll book for the next one,' I assured. 'It will give you more time to pack your case and get better than ever.'

'If I get any better than this,' he remarked drily, 'I'll be able to do it on my own. I won't need an aeroplane.'

Another blight that hit our economy at that time, was a wretched postal strike. Neither of us realised, until the mail stopped, just how many people cared about us. Every day there had been letters, asking about Martin, sending him cheery messages and news, assuring us of prayers. Charities were negotiating grants. All that was held up. Communication is vital, but no more so than where you are dependent on other people for sustenance. We despaired of the government, consoled each other with re-reading past letters, and counted the days till it ended.

Long before that though, Martin began

to lose time off school. He was very difficult to rouse in the mornings. Many a day I felt it cruelty to get him on the road, up and about, by a quarter to nine. He was already off one day a week for his injections at the hospital. Many a Monday, after the cyclophosphamide, he was too ill to move. If he started attending late in the mornings, it would hardly be worth having him on the register at all.

His work was consistently good, when he had the energy to do it. Lethargy beset him when he came home. Then one morning he awoke with pain right down his spine, and the front of his legs. He was pale and weak. It passed, and he went off to school, plucky as ever, but when he came home for lunch, he curled up on the settee and went to sleep. I didn't waken him.

He was away from school ten days. I had his homework set, and we did it together. His hands were so frail, I had to help with the writing, but his brain was alert enough. Days after that, he complained of a sore throat. He was due at the clinic, so I kept him off the rest of that week.

'Please don't tell them about my throat,' he pleaded. 'They'll keep me in hospital, I know they will.'

I felt uneasy, but by now I realised this illusion of progress was obscuring something inescapable; the existence of the original tumour. He was terrified of separation, and the alleviation of his fear was more, far more to me, than the possible development of a minor, or even a major complication. I examined his throat. There was nothing to see.

'If he asks me, I won't lie,' I said gravely. 'If he doesn't, I won't tell him.' There were a lot of sore throats about after all. It was mid-winter. It wasn't bad enough to merit an aspirin. He very soon forgot it. But the sore throat kept coming back. Lumps were coming up on his scalp that were painless but ridiculous. He didn't like it at all. Very sensitive about his appearance, he hated anything that singled him out, and couldn't bear to be ridiculed. Fortunately, his hair hid them so nobody knew. I minimised them and took his attention away. 'Just the drugs love. When they stop, the lumps will go.' It was true.

The leg pains were getting worse, and more frequent. I didn't dare to think why. When his spine started up too, it went into spasms; he went like a stiff comma that couldn't uncurl. I just put him to bed and stayed with him, holding a hand. He was red and wretched and crotchety under his cross. He resented it wearily. I gave him tablets and waited with him till it was gone, then gave him something new and novel to do, making him forget. All the time my mind worked on 'Why?', and what caused the pain and how we could prevent it from happening again.

The minute he was over these spasms, it was up and back to living again. I would not let him see himself as an invalid. He had an easily deflated nature, now, and fell speedily to gloom. I dispelled it at command and set him on his feet again. I had seen so many patients, older it is true, go down under death long before it was due, out of sheer lack of will to live. It didn't help them, and it made life a misery for those around them. While you're alive you have to live.

All the same, I begrudged the time he was away from me, studying at school for a career he may never see. I couldn't settle at home, while he was away there, wondering how he was coping. Eventually, of course, we had to admit he wasn't. I had to see Sister and explain. 'It doesn't matter,' she said gently, with a look that met mine in complete understanding. He was such an eager, obedient, good and appealing child, and she loved him too. 'Just send him when he wants to come. Don't let him worry about anything.' He could not have been in a better place, surrounded by faith and love and informality. But we both knew, Sister and I, that it could not go on this way. His days with her were numbered.

CHAPTER 10

Set-back

February saw the court case over, and my good name cleared. I was declared 'not guilty' of any crime. It meant I could take up all the old activities again and maybe make a start earning us out of debt. We were booked for Lourdes, and now had money to raise for the pilgrimage, plus incidental expenses.

Early in March, Martin came in declaring cheerfully that he had mumps. I chaffed at the idea. I had enough without that. But washing his face that night, I discovered there certainly was a swelling, just under the left side of his jaw. On palpation, I could feel similar lumps to the ones he had on his head. I made a mental, unemotional note; this was something that simply could not be overlooked.

To be honest, Martin was not the most compelling member of the household at that time. He had his bad days, that we all knew and accepted. What mattered was keeping the whole unit organised and everybody cared for. He was just one of the family. When he needed me, I was there. When he could manage, I gave much-needed attention to one of the others. There was always too much to do, and never a day's relief. I had no time to sit down and weep over what might be only swollen glands. He wasn't in any pain, and we were due for his check-up in a week. Whatever it was could wait. But I kept him off school.

The stairs were proving a nuisance now, and I had taken to carrying him up at night. There never seemed to be anybody around. It was the quickest, and the safest. He tried, when he could, to do it on his own, but I couldn't bear his unselfishness at times. What point was there in exercising to the point of pain? I was usually in a hurry and the obvious was to pick him up. Consequently I ricked my back.

It was around that time I took him, and the rest of the children, to see 'Trial by Jury'. He was interested in music, enjoyed rhythm, and I wanted to introduce him to Gilbert and Sullivan. Everywhere we went he writhed in his seat. He could never sit still for long. That afternoon, I was restless too, unable to find a position in which my spine was comfortable. The performance was a penance for me. But it gave me a new insight into Martin's condition, and his character. How long had he suffered like this, long before we knew what was wrong with him, when they commented irritably on his restlessness? They had to be made to understand.

The day we went to the clinic, the consultant looked gravely at Martin's jaw. I had to point it out, and did so silently, over Martin's head. He said solemly that the child would have to be admitted to hospital, for an 'investigation'. It was quite obvious, though neither of us said so, secondaries had sprouted in his neck. I knew it. I knew it as soon as I saw it. I just knew also that there was nothing could be done, except to make him suffer more. The treatment was as bad as the disease.

Martin broke down utterly and completely. He sobbed in the surgeon's office as though it were all my fault and all I had to do was refuse, to make him happy again. It had to be done. There had to be a biopsy. But we were going to Lourdes first. I needed a break. I wasn't strong enough to face this new development. My spirit was failing. So much disappointment after so much hope, I was defeated.

We argued a little. Taking a child out of the country, in that condition, seemed irrelevant and unnecessary. I knew what it meant to Martin, to be deprived of this again. We couldn't alter the date of the pilgrimage. I also knew that if we didn't go now, he may never make it. He was deteriorating rapidly. I insisted. The surgeon agreed. Martin could go to Lourdes, but be admitted to hospital for the exploratory examination immediately he arrived home. I told him the good, and made him utterly forget the bad. It was not going to spoil the present. 'Think about France Martin,' I urged him on the way. 'Think about the aeroplane and the train. By the time we get back, you may not need the operation.' I wasn't lying, they might, at that, decide it was unnecessary.

They didn't, and my little plan was defeated. We had a letter to say the surgeon was going away and Martin would have to have the biopsy *before* leaving for Lourdes. So he was jostled into hospital, one Sunday afternoon, and I left him looking very resentful indeed. I had taken him everything possible to keep his mind occupied. He was just geared against living another way than the one we had put together ourselves. Away from me, among strangers, he was insecure and afraid.

That night I went to bed at eight, and slept till seven. So many nights had been disturbed by Martin's pain. I hadn't had a day free of his needs in weeks. This new blow was a positive physical burden.

More treatment. More tedious journeys. More sitting around hospital waiting rooms, wasting life away. The ambulances, by then, were on a go-slow, for higher wages. Three hours was nothing to sit around, just waiting, and so much to be done at home. It was all incredibly frustrating, and exhausting in the extreme. Other children could not be left indefinitely. There was nobody else I could send Martin with. Life seemed utterly and completely impossible.

Just before he went into hospital, I took him to an Irish Feis in the school hall. It was a wet day. He couldn't walk, nor could I by then. The Saturday morning shopping was enough to finish me. We took a taxi; a mad extravagance. The hall was full of noise; so many children he knew. He had been away from them too long, though, and there was a shyness. The relationships were leaving him. He wasn't conscious of any crisis coming. He had done as I said, and just put the whole of life to one side to concentrate on the present, which was the music, the dancing, the crisps, lemonade, bags of sweets and noise. He was as happy as a boy can be, protected from reality.

I remember I sat and looked at him, with his little lumpy face all lit up with excitement. I didn't want him ever to be anything else, but just like that, completely untouched by life. There was a preciousness about him; an illumination in his spirit. How long was I going to be able to keep him this way. How long, O Lord, how long? His face was so tiny, for such a disease. I had seen what it could do. These glands affected now were pitifully, dangerously near so many vital senses; his ears, his eyes, his breathing, and his brain.

'Please God,' I prayed, with a falter, as everything that was a mother wept in me. 'Please God don't let him ever realise. Don't let him ever know.'

I brought them all home in a spirit of complete and utter despair. It wasn't any use. I couldn't do it. I'd taken on too much, and I was beaten. Somebody else would have to take Martin and make him happy. I'd had enough. What with poverty, the loneliness, the strain of looking after all the others, so many officials with entry into my home, I felt I was just a number on a file life had stamped and put in a drawer. We were nobodies; non-entities. We didn't matter.

It is possible to suffer so much that you lose faith, in God, yourself and all humanity. Mine was in dire need of a change of climate and good Spring shower.

CHAPTER 11

Thrill of a life-time

The colossal responsibility of taking a sick child 1,000 miles on my own didn't hit me till we were really on the way. We boarded a bus from the end of the street to the station, waving happy hands to those we were leaving behind. It was ten at night and a jet streaked overhead flicking night-lights in a thrilling promise. 'Maybe we will be hi-jacked,' Martin said eagerly.

I sat, breathless, watching, his pale, intense expression, this thin frame cuddled by a new duffle coat, and realised just what I was doing. A boy in an advanced state of cancer, still in weak shock from the latest development; a boy unable to lie, or sit, stand or walk for long. A boy subject to fierce, crippling attacks of pain. He'd already had four days of radium treatment to his face and neck, which could produce uneasy side-effects. We had two suit-cases, complicated documents, five stages to each journey, each way, and I'd never been up in the air before. Supposing..? Oh, what was the use of speculating? Whatever happened we'd take it as it came.

He was in high spirits, despite his swollen face. Being released from hospital was a tonic in itself. He'd had a dizzy half-day before we left, busy as a jumping-jack, packing his case, making quick visits. His school class had made a voluntary collection. The lady newsagent who kept his comics, and had herself lost a child, gave him 50p. There was more than money in that gift. The home 'Lourdes fund' had been emptied and he obviously felt like a multi-millionaire. It all seemed so much more in francs.

As for myself, relieved of all domestic strain and noise, I was free to devote myself to him. We'd always been good company. Now we really enjoyed it. We were going to savour every golden minute.

Martin had never been a sleeper. The tiny compartment had two bunks, a fold-away sink and a hidden mirror. We investigated everything with excited intelligence. Martin tried all the lights, had a drink and a snack, then climbed up into the top bunk to sleep until London. Just outside Newcastle he climbed down again and got in beside me. 'It isn't that I'm scared,' he said practically, 'I just felt I'd like to know where you are.' He slept at my feet, soundly. I lay and savoured the freedom and prayed.

We had breakfast on a tray at five, and then sped in a taxi through dim, deserted streets to the Byzantine dignity of Westminster Cathedral; to meet the others. We were early and caught it just opening, so we had time to look around, our steps clattering cheekily through hallowed alabaster, marble and mosaic.

'It's spooky,' was Martin's holiest comment.

In one chapel there's a pelican; ancient symbol of the Blessed Sacrament. That mother bird has such devotion to her young that she will bleed herself to nourish them. I knew how she felt. Nearer the door, in St George's Chapel, lies the spare, fully-dressed body of a Saint and a hero, John Southworth. One of the British nobility who risked his life nursing fetid victims of the London plague, then was hanged, drawn and quartered at Marble Arch for the crime of being a priest. He put conscience before the State and died for liberty. Our liberty.

Two emancipated looked on the emaciated and Martin muttered, 'Oh Mam, that's horrible. Let's go.'

Further on, in the Lady Chapel, is the Latin inscription 'We fly to thy patronage O Holy Mother of God, despise not our prayers in our necessities'. We did indeed fly to her, from Gatwick two hours later, and the only thing that bothered Martin was whether he'd be able to hear pop music in French on his transistor. The take-off had been, for me, the source of many a nightmare. Martin told me not to be daft, there was nothing to it. All the same, as we lifted up off the runway and I felt the panicky need to thrust my legs through the floor to get back on to solid earth, he let out a deep breath, and admitted, 'Whew, that was windy.'

Clouds floated by the window, so close we could have touched them. The ground beneath us was a page from a school atlas. We wondered why it took the plane so long to cross it. Coming down he felt sickly, but it soon passed when he found himself in Tarbes airport surrounded by foreigners. We both had a little French; also school variety, but couldn't make out a word. He hadn't been allowed to use his radio on the plane, so all the way to Lourdes on the bus he was getting ecstatically re-acquainted. I always knew where Martin was by the music on the transistor; in a house or on a tarmac it was better than a bell on a cow.

Lourdes defies description. You couldn't put Heaven in a travelogue. All you can do is give yourself to it, and let Mary tell you why you came. It was cold when we arrived, with a light drizzle. Clambering stiffly from the bus, all we felt was exhilarating air. All we saw was the magnificent mountain. All we heard was the toy-timbred clock and typical Pyrrenaean bell. All Martin could say was 'When can we go to the shops?'

He'd never stayed in an Hotel before. Ours was near the disused dungeon where St Bernadette had lived, in abject poverty. Martin counted his francs, played with the wall lights, wallowed in luxury and was innocently, honestly amused by the French bidet. Every time I missed him he was exercising the lift. Such affluence, and I'm sure the Saint approved. She knew the hard-won virtue of being cheerful in all circumstances.

The group we joined up with had come to do an All-night Vigil for World Peace, the Church under persecution and Christian Unity. They immediately undertook to pray for Martin too, but he was excused the Vigil because of his illness. The first place we all went was the Grotto, where Martin really was under its spell. Awed and quieted, impressed by the utter peace, his eyes took in the flickering splashes of colour, the rock worn smooth by millions of pious lips, the fervent, ardent love of those present for this place. Without any instigation or instruction from me, he went down, lifted his lumpy little face, and prayed.

Once away from there, he was the complete boy-tourist. He avidly filled his bottle at the water-taps, never thinking to bathe his face. He cried off the Baths and I didn't blame him; it was cold and he wouldn't understand. He was much less impressed by the spot where Bernadette actually knelt throughout the Apparitions, than by the great candles, some six feet high and thick as trees, all spattering and spitting holy fire in stands as big as market-stalls. He spent a good half-hour earnestly going around straightening them so the grease wouldn't make such a mess.

I took him to see the stone, benign figure of Saint John Vianney, my personal patron, and Confessor de luxe; the visual aid for Parish Priests. Martin was suitably interested and impressed, absorbed the story, then when it was finished looked at me with the air of the patient pushed to a generous extreme and asked, 'NOW can we go to the shops?'

Such an excursion in the town of Lourdes, outside the Domain, is a strictly business enterprise. Inside, where the heart of the Church beats, no commerce can interfere. Its pulse is simple piety. The other side of the wall there has built up a thriving industry for people like us who want to take back evidence that we have been. You have to keep a shrewd eye on your shopping and a tight fist on the francs.

It seems to stand to reason, and business acumen, that the goods in shops near the Domain, where crowds tend to concentrate, will be more expensive than those in remote cobbled streets, but that isn't so. To be absolutely sure of a bargain you have to tour the town. So we did, and he wouldn't spend a cent until he had argued and haggled with himself till he was absolutely sure. We gradually accumulated everything from a badge for his duffle-coat, to a musical box playing the Lourdes hymn for his brother. In between was a picture of the Grotto for the school, and one for me, an assortment of medals and mementoes plus a record, in Italian, of the Lourdes processions. He decided against a cute little Tyrolean clock he really wanted because it would have taken all the rest of his money.

With all this, we collapsed in a cafe and drank cafe-au-lait at 1 franc 40c a time in cups as big as basins. The price was important. We were now poor as Bernadette. He was looking tired, and his leg was beginning to drag, and I had one more call to make. I knew one of the nuns at the nearby Hospital de Sept Doulours. I'd left a case there on my previous pilgrimage, intending to come back and do some voluntary nursing. I wanted to collect it, and decided to borrow a wheelchair for Martin.

Sister was extremely gentle, showering Martin with excited French endearment that was completely lost on him. She fetched the case then took us into the yard to find something on wheels. Martin followed but when he saw what she had in mind he turned on me in wide-eyed horror. 'I'm not going in that...PRAM!' he exploded. Sister had entirely mistaken my English and was pulling out one of the huge, hooded voitures on a high Victorian chassis in which the paralysed are pushed to the Domain. Quickly, I spotted something smaller and neater, if not in very good condition, hitched Martin into it and took to the road, thanking Sister profusely in pigeon-French and assuring her it *was* good enough, and it really was what we wanted.

We giggled all the way to the Rue Baron du Prat. They don't use wheelchairs very much in Lourdes. Pilgrims tend to bring their own. This one had wheels that were set on going in opposing directions and was virtually impossible to keep straight. That aside, I hadn't yet mastered the continental Highway Code. The course was uphill and somewhat hilarious.

That night he ate as I hadn't seen him eat in months; all sorts of things he would have refused at home. He sat among strangers, and struck up a deep friendship with a Monsignor from Africa who, we learned, was on pure pilgrimage, and had nothing at all to spend. Martin insisted on giving him something of ours, at which the priest was most humbly moved, and proud. To him, the suffering were V.I.P.s and he valued the notice of a child. Martin's other heroes were the Spiritual Director of the group; a man of great faith and humanity, plus wide experience of tragedy, and Gerry, a man in a wheelchair, with great patience.

I wanted Martiin to see Lourdes at night, so just before he went to bed I wheeled him out, down the hill again. It was a fairyland, the medieval Chateau Fort floodlit on the hill; the streets so calm and still. Out of this world, which is a very good place to be when the world is all too real.

We reached the entrance to the Domain, where our friends were keeping watch. At the gate were St Michael, triumphant over the devil and sin, Gabriel of the Anunciation, Raphael the protector of pilgrims. We bade the archangels good night, turned back and left them to do our Vigil for us. Lourdes is for prayer and penance. Martin was doing enough penance, and had never needed to be exhorted to pray. Prayer and penance banish evil. So do joy and unity. We had them all. Our wills were utterly in union with the will of God. All we wanted was a way to live it. Meantime, we were happy.

Sunday morning we were out by daybreak, peering at shuttered shops, so full of what we had in England but with a French label. We went to Mass in the parish church, then bought some long French bread and croissants to take home. Later, there was a bus ride to Bartres, unaltered since Bernadette tended sheep there over 100 years ago. It was nearly time to leave for England again before I had time to myself. I left Martin with Gerry and went to my Mother alone.

I chose the Rosary Basilica because it is larger and easier to find a space. The great mosaic of the Mother of God in the ceiling, with her arms wide to the world, and her wonderful smile, had special significance for me. Once before she had sent me back with the will to persevere. Would she do it now? How to carry these heavy crosses of life, of which Martin was only one? Whether to let him go and the institutions have him; whether to fight for our right to be together.

I know not what Mother divine did to my mind, but by the time Martin came in looking for me, I was absolutely sure. Nothing and nobody was going to take this child from me, till God did it himself. He was mine, under God. He wanted to be with me, and I loved him as nobody did. Love is powerful medicine. He wasn't the same boy, separated from me. Parting, for me, was agony.

We had our photographs taken, then just 24 hours after arriving in Lourdes, we were back at the Grotto saying goodbye. My vocation renewed, I heard the

Chaplain telling us of a woman who came to Lourdes with an incurable disease. There was no miraculous cure. Some time later her husband came back, at his wife's injunction, to say thank you, and was asked why. Mary, he said, had taught that woman how to die.

Clutching Martin close, from behind his chair, I listened. Came a sudden compelling call in me. Martin was not going to die. He was going to live. Martin was going to be cured. Not here, but back home. We were going to fight, and we were going to win. The vision touched my soul and inflamed my spirit. He was not going to die. One day *we'd* come back again, and he'd be running about like other boys. Our faith would make him whole.

It was so contrary to what the priest was saying, and took such hold on my conscious mind, there could be no doubt as to its source. The Mother of mothers was telling me, Martin was going to live. I cried quietly as I held him, and those around could not but think it was tears of sad knowledge in me. But it was a weep of joy and I told nobody. Only Martin, I confided it to him, as we pushed back to the Hotel. He said, quietly 'I know.' He'd never doubted it. I was the one who had lost faith; in God, in life and in myself.

Just before the bus left, we decided he could get the clock after all. The francs also ran to a wall-plaque for my keys, with a graceful figure of Mary and a greeting 'God Bless our Home'. Home and faith were his security, and his hope. I vowed again that nobody would take them from him.

On the flight back, there was much gaiety and swopping of addresses. The pilot let Martin go up beside him, part of the way, adding to the joy in him. Later there was a shower, the question of a storm, and then it passed and the sun came through. I looked idly out and said 'Oh Martin, look!' Over to the east, over Lourdes, central in the heavens, was a rainbow, formed in an oval, radiating light. 'The Miraculous Medal,' he gasped.

It was one familiar to us, that he always wore. Mary's promise. We all saw it: nature plays a daughter's tricks under that Woman's hand. History is littered with them. That put a seal on her message for us. We never ceased to believe it.

Four million people a year don't go to Lourdes for no reason. They all get something. Often they don't realise till after they get home, just where the answer came. Provided they have gone in faith and true humility, they all encounter the supernatural. They all yearn to return. We went out of season, before the first of the great organised pilgrimages from all over the world. He received the Blessing of the Sick on a cold, grey afternoon, amid a group of blind Parisians chanting 'Lord, that I may see.' He never saw the vast crowds with skins of all colours, the breathtaking processions. He missed the swelling music of thousands throwing their allegiance to God, and a lot of what could be termed tourist attraction. The result was a completely unemotional rebirth of faith, enough to make a plane take off unaided. In Lourdes he was a different boy; at ease, happy and free. There was no greyness in his disposition, no trace of the sickness that had hung over him for months. No public insensitivity to his handicap, no being shoved aside by a society that didn't care. He was loved, accepted, honoured and privileged *because* he was weak. The sick are the centre of everything in Lourdes.

I did have a small physical miracle of my own, though it will never be recognised by the Medical Bureau. One of my fingers had been injured in the furniture removal. It had a useless tendon and was constantly, painfully inflamed. The Infirmary had tried everything, but it remained a troublesome nuisance, interfering with all manual work that I did. From the moment I put it in the water at Lourdes, the swelling and redness left, also the pain. They haven't returned. I can use the finger normally. I'm left with a very slight, natural deformity that gives me no trouble.

When Martin went to Lourdes, he fully

intended taking notes and writing an article for the Diocesan newspaper. He was good at English and had a bright mind for detail. It was agreed readers would be interested to know how that famous shrine looked, through the eyes of a child. When I came to empty his case at home, I found the note-book, clean and naked as the day it was bought. 'Martin,' I asked, wondering just what impression had been left that was worth publishing. 'What did you think of Lourdes?'

He looked up from what he was doing, smiled absently, and shook his head in a complete inability to express himself. Then he did find expression in the most profound appreciation he knew. 'It was GREAT.'

That's Lourdes.

CHAPTER 12

The miracle

The first thing that happens to faith is a testing. What we believed was neither stupid nor unprecedented. Cures of even advanced cancer are recorded, and not only in Lourdes. Daily we seemed to read reports of a new advance in research, or the personal testimony of someone who had recovered. I didn't look into any of these too closely. I just believed it wasn't possible.

Martin went straight back into hospital after our weekend away, and immediately all his symptoms returned. It was as though, like the Red Sea held back for the chariots to pass, our troubles had been at bay. From being full of 'go' on the journey home, he came to a full stop in hospital.

I visited him that afternoon and couldn't believe he was the same boy. His face was badly swollen, his eyelids streaked yellow and red. His neck was so sore they'd had to give him pain-killer, and he wouldn't eat or drink. He was very unhappy.

Tired and dispirited myself, I sat by his bed and tried to cheer him. He was very attached to his puppets, and a new one had arrived that morning; a lovely surprise. He'd had one given for Christmas that positively frightened him with its evil witch's face. I didn't care for it either. Just before the postal strike, I'd returned it to the manufacturer, explaining about Martin's illness, and reaction. Now, weeks later, they were able to send a replacement; a bright red soldier. He eyed it, and he was pleased, but there was an underlying lack of response. So I quickly made up a story; a play we could enact with all the puppets he had, when he came home.

The other children had sent him messages; comics, get-well cards and instructions to 'hurry home'. That was just the trouble, and no medicine could cure it. The boy was homesick. He'd had his radium for that day; fifteen minutes at the Infirmary across the town. He was able to walk. So I asked permission to take him out for an hour. That brought him back to normal.

I was pushed for time. Another mother had generously taken the two younger boys for the weekend. I had to meet them from school. I left Martin, tucked up in bed, submerged again in his gloom. Life was all raw and disappointing.

Next day they let me take him for his treatment; partly to relieve the staff. The ambulance was very late. I had left everything at home. I was chafing at precious time passing. The other adult patients travelling *would* try to be friendly, which was helpful normally, but now they all wanted to know what was wrong with Martin. In front of the child, I couldn't tell them. The pressure on my powers of invention I found a trial. Martin was too ill to talk, and they wouldn't leave him alone.

The Radiology Department, despite the light paint, was the most depressing place we had ever been in. It had its own distinctive metallic smell that hit us as we went in. All the victims had the same silent air of despair and fatalistic dying. It is no place for a child. I took him out of the waiting-room and sat with him in the corridor. Another wait.

On the way back, he began to cry. 'I wish we didn't have to come back here...'

'Oh love, don't,' I pleaded. 'You'll only be in hospital a few days...'

'A few *days!*' he wailed. 'But they're not *doing* anything!'

That was true. When I got back to the ward, I asked if he couldn't be discharged and have his treatment as an outpatient. After some haggling, the specialist was approached and he agreed. I could take him home, if I undertook to have him at the Infirmary for radium every day except Saturday and Sunday, then back at that hospital for his injection on Friday.

It was a heavy undertaking. I had a

three-storey house and five others to cook, clean and shop for. But just to see Martin's face left no hesitation in me. He positively leaped out of that ward, waving cheery goodbyes, completely his old self again.

How valuable is privacy when you are living secret tragedy. The ambulance journeys got worse. The wages dispute was still on; some of the men treated us as though it were our fault they had to work at all. I never knew what time they were coming, or how long we'd have to wait. One day it took us four hours to get him his fifteen minutes treatment, and we lived two miles from the Infirmary.

Part of the semi-strike was that the men would agree to run the ambulances, but they would do nothing for the patients. Martin was getting progressively weaker. I had to lift him in and out myself, with great muscular men looking on. I also went to assist arthritic cripples, whose clinic was on our route. It was the disgust at human nature that sickened me as much as the waste of time.

Martin didn't mind the treatment. It was painless. In the room itself, the girls were friendly and kind. He'd brought them a card from Lourdes and they stuck in on the door. For the fifteen minutes he lay on the couch with his transistor in his ear, taking his mind off the environment.

At home, he was eating fairly well, though is sickness persisted and was getting worse. He had appetite, but if he satisfied it, his system rebelled. He was also getting progressively drowsy. On the day he had to attend two different clinics, I found it difficult to rouse him. He was heavy and feeling so ill I had to wash and dress him myself, then carry him like a baby down two curving flights of stairs. Before the radium, he vomited copiously. He pulled round, and we took a taxi on to the hospital for his injection. He was too ill to travel by ambulance.

We arrived to find the clinic finished and the doctor gone. They found him, but then the drug was missing. Another wait. Martin tried hard to pull himself together, terrified the doctor would say he had to be admitted. It was late afternoon when I got him home and he wasn't the only one on the cliff of collapse. That day I vowed we would cut free of the State system. The next week I took him in by taxi. The whole thing was over in an hour.

During the weekend between though, he deteriorated rapidly. Saturday he was vomiting bile from very early in the day. His eyes were puffed up and discoloured; his features Mongolian. He couldn't get even Lourdes water past his mouth. He had a headache he said.

Sunday he was limp and drowsy, the veins in his scalp blue and distended. His whole head was 'sore inside'. I gave him tablets but he vomited them back. His leg was hurting and I couldn't relieve that either, except with a hot water bottle, which he found such a relief I had to fill it every three hours. His swollen abdomen was painful. He couldn't sit up properly. He was very much aware that he had been in bed for two days and was determined to throw it off. *He* wasn't going to be ill, he said.

Next day, Monday, that treatment began again, now increased to thirty minutes. The inside of his mouth, on the left side, was raw and peeling. It was slow going. His every movement was an effort, for both of us.

When we got home I found him strangely lacking in attention to what I was saying. He just sat about, or lay down, and didn't seem to know when I was there. Then I caught him impatiently shaking his transistor. 'Something wrong?', I asked.

'It isn't working.'

'Oh give it to me. Probably the batteries. I'll get you a new lot.' Just before going to the shop, I checked, just in case he had given it a knock and really done it an injury. There was nothing wrong with the transistor radio. It was Martin. He couldn't hear.

Later that day, the doctor from the hospital where he had his injection rang to say that his blood count was down; alarmingly low. He'd have to have a test taken, the next day. Suddenly the whole thing became clear to me. What was obviously happening was that too many cell-destroying agents were being poured into the child and his normal cells were being adversely affected. It was ridiculous, but fairly common-place in cancer therapy. They are fighting for life and aim at killing the malignancy.

Next day Martin was very droopy, and cried easily, but still kept fighting it off. I had a brief television recording I couldn't cancel, and he desperately pleaded to come. He did so enjoy it, and he obviously did want to feel part of life, not an invalid. We took a taxi both ways. It was over in a very short time, but Martin could hardly keep his eyes open. Only then did I begin to realise that this drowsiness was not tiredness, but something very much worse.

Really alarmed, I got him home and up on to the settee in my room. That way he felt privileged, not ill. I left him there, fully clothed, and went to organise the others. Every time I went back to him, he opened his eyes, and he moved, but he didn't want to get up at all.

I intended staying awake with him all that night, but I was utterly exhausted and kept dozing off. At daybreak, when I went over to him, he was exactly as I had left him and he didn't move when I shook him. This wasn't sleep. It was a coma.

Quickly I got the family up, fed and out to school, then took him straight to the Infirmary. As he'd roused slightly, he was bringing up great gulps of frothy yellow fluid. His thirst was insatiable, and no wonder. He couldn't keep anything down. He had no pain, but nor had he any sensation. His reflexes were numb. All he did when his glazed eyes rolled open was to look around for me.

The radiologist was sent for, took one look and shook his head. 'It's obviously working under his skull.'

Whether he meant the cancer or the radium I didn't stop to ask. By then I was fully decided this was the end of the line as far as their methods were concerned. They'd done their best, very much against my instinct. It seemed they were succeeding. Then it was obvious they weren't. The drugs hadn't stopped secondaries from sprouting, and the radium hadn't prevented this.

The radiologist was murmuring something about 'Get him admitted...' when everything in me broke into revolt. 'No,' I almost shrieked. I steadied myself under fatigue and considerable duress to tell him clearly. 'There isn't anybody, anywhere, who can look after him as well as I can. He'll die in here. There isn't anything more you can do.'

He shrugged, unwillingly. 'Very well. If you think you can...'

'I'll manage.' I rang a taxi and took Martin away, out of medical care. I took him home and carried him, alone, up to the top floor to my bed. Then I rang the Presbytery, told the priest what had happened, and asked him to come. We still had one other authority to consult. God is the arbiter of life, and I wanted his verdict.

It was Maundy Thursday. The priests

were up to their dog-collars in Holy Week ceremonies, but two of them promised to come. One, the younger, had just been ordained and this was his first such call. We had the water from Lourdes, a Rosary, hand-made for Martin by a man we had never met. There was the plaque on the wall, 'God Bless Our Home'. Faith was all we had left.

Martin was grey and swollen, moving only to spurt out foul yellow froth, to the moment before the first priest arrived. The child couldn't speak to make the responses, so I did it for him. What bothered me most was that even if he managed to swallow the water at Communion, he would certainly not be able to keep it down. I warned the priest, and he decided to wait until the time came and see what happened.

The time came. 'Martin,' I whispered gently in his ear. 'Communion love.' I slipped an arm behind his shoulders, and he sat up. He opened his mouth, took the host with his tongue, followed by enough water to swill it down. Then he lay back and went into stupor again.

The other priest came to anoint him. The limp limbs had to be lifted, each in turn. I held hard on to the side of the bed and appealed, 'Please God, spare him. Don't let him be sick. I do believe.'

I did too. That was the lunatic thing. I really did think this crisis would pass. Even though I knew how far the disease had gone. Even though, downstairs on the step, the priest consoled and said, 'He hasn't long.' He had seen death, and death like this, but he was just a man. A wise, kind, experienced, intelligent man. But just a man. He wasn't God.

I went back to Martin's room and cleared away. The other children were all watching television. They knew there was some cause for concern, but weren't unduly perturbed. I sat and waited.

Martin was anointed at exactly ten minutes past six. At twenty minutes to seven, he turned his head and said 'Mam, where's my transistor?'

I put it near his ear. He smiled, slowly. 'That's better. It's working all right now.'

He could hear.

I waited, till he said suddenly, more urgently, 'What time is it?'

'Nearly seven o'clock.'

'Oh Mam,' reproachfully. 'I'm missing all the good programmes. Get me up. I want to go downstairs.'

Without protest, I got him his dressing gown and slippers, and carried him down. He wanted nothing to eat, but drank easily, naturally, and kept the fluid in him. There was no sickness or even nausea. It was nine o'clock before he said he was tired and wanted to go back to bed. He slept all night, and it was natural sleep. We were both undisturbed. I was so sure, by then, that I went to bed myself and didn't even watch him.

Medicine and religion tend to be thought incompatible. They do in fact, make a fine working partnership, but not if the rights and ideals of each are set at war on one another by the ignorant or partisan, and not if we forget that God is in charge of both. His rights are supreme. He still has the power to take the forces of nature and subdue them to His own will.

I wasn't foolish enought to presume Martin cured. He obviously wasn't. He still had his great swollen tummy and the growth inside his mouth. But the brain symptoms had vanished, and never did return. His face didn't hurt him again on that side; it remained quiescent, and from the moment he received Communion, he was never sick again. God spared him to eat and enjoy his food, provided we were sensible, until the very end.

As for me, the course ahead was clear. God had spoken. 'Hope on. Believe on. I am here. Do not despair.'

CHAPTER 13

Spared

On Good Friday morning, he woke early, and was straight up out of bed. He wanted to be dressed. We had some other children staying, as arranged before we knew what crisis was going to hit us. By nine o'clock they were all downstairs hilariously playing cards and drinking coffee.

'Anything you want love?' I asked him, having a quick check before taking a note around to the Presbytery.

'Iced lollies,' he said cheerfully, slapping down an ace. 'My mouth is stiff.'

It wasn't so stiff he couldn't giggle. He was sunny and bright as the spring morning coming to life outside. The puffiness was almost gone from around his eyes.

I boarded the bicycle, spun round the

parish, and found a shop doing early Bank Holiday trade; an ever-open store run by Pakistanis. I came back with a feast, not exactly befitting the solemnity of the day, but God surely approved. Our Resurrection had come a little early.

Later that morning, I found the house empty. The children had all gone down to the Valley to play; Martin included. He was one of them again. When he came back he was tired, but he'd walked further than he had been able to go in weeks. I sat them all outside the house for lunch.

Round the corner, the nuns from the school had been informed of Martin's rapid decline, and the fact that he was being anointed. I hadn't had a chance, because of their morning devotions, to tell them the news, so had to laugh when two of them rounded the corner, anxiously coming to comfort the dying, and maybe the bereaved. There they found the child, far from moribund, sitting in a deckchair eating fish and chips! They listened, amazed, gave Martin their love, then hurried back, full, to tell the others; two women at the sepulchre, seeing Christ on Easter day.

Saturday the reaction set in. Martin had survived what could have felled a healthy adult. His energy was more determination than strength and he needed rest, but he woke up at eight and got up, hardly able to totter. He sat by the fire in my attic, and would not give in. Bed was for illness and he wasn't ill.

Anxiously I sought my mind for something to give him sense. I knew what the trouble was. He was afraid if he didn't hang on to this improvement, life-line that it was, he would lose it. The fear made him panicky, and irritable.

Then I remembered. It was only Saturday, not Easter yet, for the others anyway, but we were on God's schedule, and could bend.

'Would you like your Easter egg?' I asked.

His face said, 'Ugh,' chocolate had had no appeal for him for many a month. But his kind little mind and generous soul said, patiently, 'If you like.'

I felt in a carrier at the bottom of the wardrobe and brought it out; large, blue as the sky and the mantle of the Virgin. 'A present from Our Lady,' I said, and handed it to him.

He took the box in wonder, undid the bow, and lifted off the lid. Inside, cuddled by tissue, was a watch; man size, with a blue dial, a striped strap, and the date. I'd dashed out and bought it, on an inspiration, just a few days before, when he was so depressed. Hours later I'd wondered if he'd ever see it. Now there it was, the answer to a fervent prayer, magnificently timed.

'It's just what I wanted,' he breathed, too weary to get excited. But the tension had gone out of him. His face had cleared. 'You said I could have it for Christmas,' he reminded.

'Oh well, you know me. I haven't got a watch and *somebody* in the house has to be able to tell me the time.'

He smiled. The house was silent. I suggested he went back to bed. He went without a murmur. He lay listening to the tick of it, now and again glancing down at the dial. Bemused happiness. Peace. Faith revived. He went off to sleep and didn't wake again until eleven.

Just one little incident marred that day, as his energy returned. His hair, as he groomed it, seemed to be dropping out. 'Hey, look at that,' he said, alarmed, showing me the comb. He was highly sensitive about his appearance.

'Oh, that isn't much,' I argued. 'That happens to me too.' But I remembered the doctor's warning, and something in me winced.

Easter Sunday, he insisted on going to Mass. A neighbour gave us all a lift. He couldn't sit upright; the old back trouble was still evident, but he leaned on the rail and saw it through. He wanted to prove himself. Not only that, as we came home, he confided. 'You know Mam, every time I go to Communion, I feel better.'

Relieved of the sickness, his appetite was becoming more adventurous. He ate chocolate and enjoyed it. He picked at everything festive, had a good lunch, then decided he'd like to go to the cinema. We all agreed. There was a new Disney epic on in town that just suited our mood. Martin walked both ways, to and from the bus. He was a film fanatic. One year, when he was eight, he'd won a painting competition that earned us two free seats to see 'Ring of Bright Water'. We'd never been in the Circle before, and sat eating chocolates as though we owned the place. Nothing ugly or adult or violent appealed to his gentle nature, but anything musical, funny or human and he was hooked.

Monday, after a slow start, we went to the Museum, into the park, and on the boats. He couldn't row but he could splash. And he could laugh. He filled himself with ice-cream, cola, coffee and nuts. There was little difference between him and all the others; only that his excitement was keener, his enjoyment deeper, and his awareness of joy more apparent.

Only one thing marred it. Over the road was the building where, up till a week ago, he had lived through so many nightmares. 'Mam,' he said, earnestly as the cloud fell on him. 'Do I have to go back to that hospital?'

His anxious eyes said, 'I'm all well now. We don't need them any more.'

I had to think. I knew the truth of his persisting condition. I didn't know the mind of God, as to its healing. It would be a serious and a solemn undertaking, to cut off completely from orthodox medicine, and yet, I knew the difference it would make to him. Just to be free, absolutely free, of injections, waiting-rooms, strong clean paint an unfamiliar faces above white coats. Not to have to waste away life in clinic boredom, with so much to be done outside. Not to be made to *feel* ill, by simply having to enter the environment of illness.

That aside, I myself longed to be free, to give my dietectic theory a chance. Cancer, I was sure, was a deficiency disease, producing auto-intoxication. The answer was systemic hygiene. How could that possibly operate in a body pumped full of drugs and radium which are in themselves poisons? What mother in her right mind would again put a child to all he had been through, without even the guarantee that he would be free of it eventually?

'No love,' I promised him 'You're not going back.'

He beamed. 'That's *great,'* and then fired another broadside on my feeling mind, 'And do I have to go back to school?'

It wasn't so much that he hadn't liked being there. I knew that. It was the strain those few weeks had been, keeping physically up to healthy boys, and the journey both ways. 'No,' I assured. 'You're on an extended holiday. Order of the nurse-in-charge. You'll go back when you can run both ways. After the summer holidays.'

He leaped off away from me to join and tell the others. He was going to enjoy life, to that I vowed, and he was going to be happy. Never again would he feel the cage of illness closing in on him. Never again would we be separated. In the vague distance I saw September; a new term and for him a new life. Six months. We had six months to beat this thing. We could. I knew we could.

Watching them playing, I did a mental meander around what had brought me to this theory, so despised in medical circles. In training I was made to think cancer is a mystery disease of unknown cause, that nothing other than surgery or radium is any use, and that if they fail the case is hopeless. Later, nursing the patients themselves, I began some independent thinking, and listening, and reading. Cancer was not new. It had been treated, and cured, before radium and without surgery. Hippocrates maintained that it was 'a general bodily disease which eventually produced a local outbreak in the form of a growth.' What caused the 'general bodily disease?' And why, in this century had it reached the proportions of a plague?

There is no cancer among primitive races living on a natural, wholesome diet. Savages had developed cancer when they adopted the eating habits of civilised people. It followed that cancer is a disease of civilisation.

Didn't I know, as a nurse trained in dietetics, how difficult it was to get what I knew to be good food, and then to get the family to eat it? We live in a society where natural goodness had been bleached or beaten out, where food faking is an industry, where dyes and preservatives are included by habit. Crops are sprayed with poision before they reach the shops. Greed for money was making people eat rubbish in pretty boxes. White sugar from birth (and before) was vitiating the national taste for natural food. White flour had everything God put into the grain, thrown away, for the sake of appearances, and texture. The result was very poor national health.

A poisoned system, deprived of oxygen, with its chemical balance gone askew, could very readily produce a fungus. Right the balance and the fungus would be attacked. A healthy body is equipped to fight. Successes are recorded, but not in the popular newspaper, and not in the orthodox journals. Anybody I knew seeing the connection between cancer and carrot juice was labelled a crank.

But I had a child for whom drugs, surgery and radium could do nothing except make him suffer more. I had every reason to withdraw from the medical scene, to treat him with common-sense and a respect for the laws of nature. It was worth a try. Surgery and radium deal with the effects. They do not tackle the cause. When they are successful, and they are for some, it is very often accompanied by a much closer attention to diet and general health by a thoroughly frightened patient. Where I had seen failure, it was often due to a conviction that death was inevitable, and lack of proper home care. The patient simply lost the will to live. Death was forced on him by a society that believe him dead already.

My treatment was impossible in hospital and for most mothers. But training, detachment and clear judgement, plus an eye for detail, were surely an asset?

I wasn't a worshipper of the god of orthodox medicine. I had seen too much innocuous hypocrisy, professional jealousy, pride, prejudice and refusal to listen. 'Official' attitudes are a mass of contradictions. Doctors are qualified in illness, not perfect health. The naturopath, homeopath, osteopath and herbalist were ridiculed as rivals and quacks. But they do relieve human suffering and they do get results. But not on the National Health. I was faced with an expensive experiment and nowhere to go for support. But I knew, as I knew my son, it was the only way. God would provide. If we had to do without everything else, we would get Martin what he needed.

One thing I didn't have to worry about was his interest in living. Sparkling and cheerful, full of zest for living, he was an ideal guinea-pig. What had we to lose?

CHAPTER 14

The treatment

I notified the hospital of my decision, without going into the reasons. I was deeply grateful to them for what they had done. It was to them I owed Martin's rescue and diagnosis. We had simply reached a stage where he either died with them or lived with me, whatever 'life' may be. I was exercising my parental right to choose what I felt to be best for my own child.

The specialist understood and sympathised. He assured me that they would always be there, if we were to need them, any time. With that safety-valve, plus God and logic, we laid out a new schedule for a child I must now regard as convalescent. I had to look on that wretched disease as already beneath us, otherwise there was no resolution. We were winning. We had it where it belonged. We'd live above it, till it was beaten underground never to rise.

Basic to the treatment was elimination of toxins, and the prevention of their build-up again, and one absolute essential was fresh air. Martin could not walk very far or very fast. On bad days, he was crippled with pain. After Easter I approached the Red Cross and they loaned us a folding wheelchair which I fondly imagined would get us out anywhere, even on a bus.

I hadn't taken into account my own frailty. Seven children had taken their toll on me, in terms of heavy lifting. I had been warned to avoid it. The chair was heavy, and Martin was no paperweight. I found it difficult to negotiate, especially up and down kerbs.

'You ought to have 'L' plates,' he protested, clinging hard on to the arms, wondering how far he could trust me.

'You criticise and you'll end up in the gutter,' I muttered. On several occasions he nearly did.

The first ride was an absolute riot, and an indication of out mutual determination to see the world. It was raining and he was bored in the house. He wanted some balsa wood up the High Street. He wanted something different to eat. Why didn't we try the chair? There wouldn't be many people about.

So in puddling rain, with a macintosh covering him, and an umbrella nearly covering me, we splashed happily from shop to shop, inspiring a wide variety of responses, from admiration, pity and compassion, to irritation, anger and contempt. We came back refreshed, exhilarated and very wet, with an addition to the health regime.

Potassium I knew to be vital, and missing from modern feeding. It controls the grey matter of the brain, and thus ties up with anxiety. I knew cancer to be associated with mental stress. Martin's first symptoms had developed when he saw me being ill-treated by his father. Potash is also a radio-active alkali attracting oxygen to the blood. He could eat apples, but not many and not easily. That day we discovered apple juice. From unsprayed crops.

Pain was niggling him most of the time, I found, though he very seldom complained. He was so used to it, he took it as a way of life. Cancer is not in itself a painful condition. It is the site of the nerve involvement which causes pain. Martin's disease was in the soft tissues, so was not a great trial in that respect, but he did have the fluid, inflammation and pressure affecting his hip and legs, plus distension of his abdomen. A couple of headache tablets usually kept it manageable, and I never took him anywhere without them.

His hair continued to drop out, even on his pillow. In a very short time he had a bald patch that gave him great distress.

'Don't worry, it will come in again,' I assured. Now that he was off the drugs it would. He still wasn't very pleased. Eventually, to his wailing dismay, he found there was no stopping the hair leaving his head, and was left with a scalp completely bared, from a clear line going right across his skull from one ear to the other. Weeping, he pummelled his pillow and said, 'I'll never be able to go out again. Never! They'll all laugh at me. I look like a Mohican Red Indian.'

He did indeed. The first of the Mohicans. His child's face and old-man baldness made him a freak. He looked utterly ridiculous. The scalp was still covered in lumps, colourless but obvious. I tried combing the back hair over, but it wasn't long enough. It made him look worse.

'Oh Martin,' I pleaded, as grieved as he was. 'It isn't nearly as bad as losing a leg. You can wear a hat when you go out. Inside...well, they'll just have to get used to it. And they will.'

I didn't feel nearly as confident as I tried to sound. Children are tasteless, callous and cruel; no more so than when confronted by a physical disability.

He was so deeply sensitive, and reliant on their company. We had achieved normality to a great extent and now here was this marking him out as different. I knew how I felt when my hair was a mess. I wouldn't be surprised if he never went downstairs again.

He did, but he wore a hat; a wool balaclava. When the other children asked him why, he told them to 'shut up.' He was cold. He struggled with his tears, and watched television with his little face working tremulously all night. He went to bed early. After he'd gone, I explained to the others what had happened. I warned them they weren't to say a word, but to act as though he had always looked that way. Of course, all that did was arouse their curiosity. When Martin did at last brave the ordeal, it was defiantly, and there was no comment, just a tense atmosphere of strain. It was a terrible affliction, felt most of all by his pretty sister, but they would, I knew, get used to it.

Then one day I said casually to him, from behind the wheelchair when we were out. 'You know Martin, there's a comedian on television with a lot less hair than you. He's famous. Everybody loves him and he gets a lot of laughs.'

Martin didn't say anything, but next time that comedian was on screen, I made sure he saw the programme. Not long afterwards, all the children were at home one day, and I heard shrieks of laughter, coming from the dining-room. There was Martin, up on the table, in the centre of a little crowd, mimicking the comedian, pulling back what little hair he did have, to make himself look the same. 'Look at me,' he yelled, 'Look at me. Guess who I am?'

I did. Admiration surged in me, and gratitude, for his native courage, and that indefeatable sense of humour that made him see his advantage. He was one up on them. He was funnier. He could make them laugh.

The tension gone, he never again felt self-conscious at home over any indignity. He had learned to laugh at himself. He had grown up a little more. As the hair grew back, it was possible to comb it over and hide the blank expanse, to some extent. He did collect a variety of hats, only one of which he wore; a black and white peaked effort in his City football stripes. But it was plastic and on hot days it was just too much, he had to go without, I tremble still with wrath at the ignorant adults and unchecked children who made him suffer for it. Their rudeness and utter lack of concern for his feelings made my heart ache. But he took it with amazing resignation. He didn't cry or rebel, and he wasn't rude in return. Just now and again when he saw people coming, he'd say, 'Oh Ma, let's go round another way. I hate everybody staring at me.'

His lively mind, I knew, must be kept ever on the move. It must not be imprisoned in his physical cage. If it wasn't kept stimulated and occupied, he would be impossible to live with. His puppets he played with for hours, till his arms tired. We never did do the play I wrote, but it remained something to look forward to. His skill with the strings was remarkable in one so young, and his patience if they tangled, amazing.

Origami he was good at. He painted, by numbers. He collected coupons and sweet wrappers and did competitions, then wallowed in the results. For kicks, he put tiny plack plastic spiders on our dinners and sat quietly, whimsically, waiting for the screams. The day his big brother ate one by mistake, we both took an oath of silence. It was safer.

Judy the dog obligingly had puppies and gave Martin many a delight. He loved life, and saw life itself in their unsteady, soft little bodies. He had such gentle hands, and was so proud when the tiny animals went to sleep on his knee, or round his neck.

The film mania persisted. He loved the early silent movies; the precision chase and quick knockabout; the expert, talking gestures with no sound. When the others went back to school, we did the round of Chaplin, Laurel and Hardy, the unforgettable Buster Keaton.

He was entranced by comic songs, of the innocent variety, and introduced the rest to George Formby humour. Cheap, long-playing records helped him build up a collection of interests and memories. He hadn't abandoned his transistor and his Pop music, but somebody had stolen it and until we could get a new one, he was bereft.

I still did the occasional television recording, and we stayed up together till near midnight to see the outcome. One day in the studio canteen, he let me down utterly with his bouncy candour. I had just bought a hair-piece and was wearing it for the first time, hoping very much it would pass as natural. The secret was well kept, till somebody remarked on my new style, and asked outright, 'Is that your own hair?' Torn between absolute honesty and reluctance to have my privacy invaded, I was struggling for a compromise, when Martin broke in loyally, 'Of course it is.' He added in evidence, 'I was with her when she bought it!'

Television on the seeing-end side, was his salvation often when I was busy. Cut off from school, he still had the urge to learn. News of his illness reached the Public Relations Executive, who had a boy of his own, and one day there arrived a full set of booklets, timetables and maps, issued to teachers using the television programmes for schools. From then on, our schedule revolved around his 'lessons'.

The same man also fixed up an occasion that set Martin's heart thumping like a drum. One of his favourite quiz programmes was being recorded at our local studio. Martin was too young for the routine audience, but he was privately invited to watch from the production box. Queues outside and staff inside must have wondered who he was, the scrap of a boy, not very attractive to look at, who couldn't even walk upright, yet was welcomed by the hostess and P.R.O., taken to the canteen and fed, introduced to other performers and generally treated like a V.I.P. He came home exhausted, with an autographed copy of the script from the Producer and a signed picture of the compere he adored. It was a neat piece of public relations that did nobody any good commercially, as it went entirely unpublicised. But it made one little boy extremely happy, and he never forgot it. A gesture of real humanity from the heart of show business.

By Whitsun, Martin had gained a stone in weight, was eating most of what I gave him, and was having no more trouble, aside from an ejected tooth, on the affected side of his face. Further than that I did not glance. He took each day as it came and lived by the hour. Each day we made a journey to church, to that Pressence, and just sat, confirming our resolution. Sometimes, in between, I went on my own. Without it I could not live. It was the source of my energy, and my strength. To give myself to Martin in this way, I had to sacrifice everything else, including my ability to earn a living. I was still fighting for legal custody of the children. I was perpetually harassed to find money for essentials like heat and light and clothing, to say nothing of Martin's needs. We had to beg all the way.

There were the constant demands of the other children. A full night's sound sleep was unusual.

I was not by nature a heroine. Courage I had had to learn by facing fear. I was the type who needed security, and life was very insecure. Without God, and my utter trust in his overpowering insight into my situation, plus his acute knowledge of what was to come, I should very quickly have lost my stability.

We were dependent on prayer, and I knew it. We summoned help, in that respect, from all corners of the earth; from Missions in Asia, Africa and Vietnam, from hospitals, religious orders and parishes, from Anglicans, Spiritualists, Non-conformists; any denomination, as well as our own. Suffering is universal and so is belief in God. Faith was our boiler and it needed constant re-fuelling. Martin was suffering, but he had hope and he had love. Whenever he heard the priest read out his name in church for prayers, his face didn't change, but he smiled in his mind. His eyes lit from behind.

And every night we all knelt in the lounge round a candle three feet high that we had brought back from Lourdes. ‘Holy Mary, Mother of God, pray for us...’

We may not have amounted to much in the eyes of British Society, but we had friends in high places.

CHAPTER 15

Dependence

The wheelchair did indeed open up a whole new world to us, though not in terms of miles. Places I have previously had to go without Martin, saving his legs, I could now take him along. He browsed in the library, listened to people talking, enjoyed the scenery, visited my friends and was able to do his own shopping. He had a mind of his own and knew exactly what he wanted. He loved to be taken to see the nuns, in a semi-enclosed Order a mile away. They mothered him, and sustained me.

His illness must have been a puzzle and a test of credulity, to casual observers. One day he'd be seen, apparently helpless in the chair. The next he'd be boarding a bus or easing into a taxi, apparently healthy. We simply geared everything to what he was able to do, and met his immediate need. But as early summer came, it was obvious to me that he was becoming increasingly dependent on both me and the wheelchair. His life was leaning more and more on what we could make it, together, in our small environment.

One thrill we discovered by accident, when returning from the convent. At the end of our street is a railway line, with a footbridge we had to cross. We well knew the rumble of the diesel, and the picturesque landmark, set in a quiet city backwater. But this afternoon we were actually on the bridge when we saw the train coming. 'Oh wait,' Martin pleaded. 'I want to see it go underneath.'

We stood, entranced, as the muffled, velvety clank of it came rhythmically nearer, between the banks and through the honour-guard of trees. The driver was standing at the wheel. Just before he reached the bridge, he looked up, saw Martin, and lifted his hand in a cheery wave. Martin laughed, and waved to him, and the driver hooted his horn. It echoed down the line as the train thundered under our feet and disappeared.

It was a golden moment, held suspended in time. We walked back home in musing wonder. 'It was like the Railway Children,' he said at last, his little face all lit with joy. I knew a closeness to him that always struck me when we shared something as deep as this; a bond thickening and tightening by the hour. It frightened me at times. What was to become of me if...? I pushed the thought out of my mind.

From then on, every shopping excursion became a race, to see if we could get to the bridge on time. As soon as we heard the clackety-clank of the diesel, I had to do a brisk Ben Hur. If we made it, there was a mad desire to cheer, even when the driver wouldn't wave. If we didn't make it, well, there was another day.

In between, we had some hard days, and the nights began to get tiresome. The pains in his legs were getting worse. As an attack came on, and the muscles went into spasms, I gave him tablets and a warm drink, but they took a while to act. In the intervening time he screamed, as any child will. I tried holding him, moving him about, nursing him. It was no use. I might just as well have not been there.

Knowing what discomfort he suffered as routine, I was reluctant to reprimand him, but there were other people in the house. Unless the screaming was actually relieving the tension, which it can, it was quite unnecessary; exhausting for him, and agony for me. It wasn't serving any useful purpose, and he was always ashamed of himself afterwards. So one day, when I could stand no more, I got up and said firmly, 'Look. That yelling is a lot of baby noise. You know very well the pain will be gone in twenty minutes. You can watch the clock. If you can't put up with it for that long, then you're no son of mine!' And I walked out and slammed the door.

I went into the yard. I heard him yelling

from a distance, through muffling doors. I would not give in. But I prayed to every saint and martyr who ever suffered. 'Please, please, give him what he needs. I can't.' When he stopped I went back in. 'Is it gone?' I asked calmly.

'No,' he said practically. 'But it will be in four minutes time.'

I sat down and held his hand, and began to read to him. He held on to me silently. When his hand relaxed, I knew the pain was gone. His muscles were still tight as a drumskin.

After that we had no more screaming. He cried, at times, but quietly and I never left him. He knew if he wanted me to stay he'd have to be a man. But the *cause* of the pain intrigued me. This wasn't from the tumour itself. What natural element was there that kept nerves and muscles healthy, easing neuritis and fibrositis? Then it came to me. A famous woman who did a lot of public speaking had written that she took lecithin, every time she had pain in her legs. Lecithin, responsible for cellular breathing; the chief component of nerve tissue. That same day I started Martin on Lecithin capsules, four times a day. Within a week, the leg cramps were easier. After two weeks they were gone.

His back and hips continued to give him trouble. The spine was out of alignment, due to the size and site of the tumour. That was bound to be an impediment, both to blood circulation and nerve force. Drugs I was determined to avoid. They start off well, but they dope the constitution. Then the patient becomes addicted and they lose their potency. Heat was the answer, and had been for some time. He was never without a hot water bottle. When he went out in the wheelchair, we tucked it where the small of his back should have been. He leaned on it to keep it in place. Days when he couldn't sit still, it needed constant re-adjustment. We always had to be back home for a refill before it was cold.

Then he began waking in the night, in pain, and the bottle had to be filled. Then it wasn't once, but twice, and three times;

every time the bottle cooled. Nights became a revolving nightmare, and I realised what had happened; Martin was 'addicted' to the hot water bottle.

This turned our routine into chaos. I had to have sleep. The days were heavy enough without facing them red-eyed, drained and jaded, unable to think or keep steady on my feet. I explained this to him, urging that I was no use to him if I wasn't strong, and he would have to go back into hospital. I asked him would he please try to manage, at least until early morning. I gave him two tablets at night before he went to sleep, hoping that would help. Another two were on the table if he needed them.

For several nights it seemed to work, then I woke in the dark, early, to hear shuffling and clattering. I went in to his room, and there he was, standing by the bed, swaying on his feet, with the steaming kettle in one hand and a very unsteady rubber bottle in the other. He had been up like that every night, doing it himself.

I appreciated his consideration, and the

will to stay at home, but it was no use. A scalded child wasn't going to help any. I just had to move in beside him and gear myself to interrupted sleep. He chose the bottle because it was effective. He did at least go straight off to sleep again.

It had long been in my mind to visit the osteopath first recommended to me. Providence made it possible, through a kindly 'neighbour' who had also benefitted from his skill and insisted on paying the consultation fee. I wrote first, explaining Martin's advanced condition and what I was trying to do. The osteopath gave us an appointment immediately.

We had to go by taxi. I was too weary to push the chair. There was a driver in the vicinity. A man with twenty years in the business who had just set up a Limited Company. I called him and told him what I had to do. Between us, we negotiated Martin into the seat, and he refused to take the fare. He said to call him again if we ever needed him.

The osteopath was young, with supple hands. He confirmed that there was no disease of the hips or legs; the pain was due to affectation of the nerves of his back. He showed me an exercise that put gentle pressure on the tumour and got around the deformity to improve circulation.

More, much more than that, he gave me encouragement. He absolutely agreed with my theory of systemic hygiene and working on the general health. He told me later that it may be possible to loosen the tumour, thus relieving the pressure and speeding up elimination of toxins. At that time, his back was much too tender; it would only increase the pain. His final words were, 'We'll work on that as he improves.'

As he IMPROVES. It was just what I needed. Deep down I was losing heart, but here was someone who believed. It restored my faith in myself. Unfortunately, the tenderness persisted. I was grateful when, at the next appointment, the osteopath refused to let me spend any more money. I was well able to do all that could be done, myself. With Martin's co-operation, we undertook the exercises several times a day, and they did relieve him considerably.

With vital exercise in mind, I had been looking for a bicycle that he could manage. On good days, it would invigorate his circulation and add zest to life. I scoured the town and found one, reduced as shop-soiled. His sister and I collected it, unknown to him, and walked it the three miles home. He was very depressed that day, and we'd left him sleeping on the settee. When he opened his eyes, not very happily, there was this magnificent machine, shining red, white and blue, complete with bag, tools and inflator. His face lit, and his spirit leaped to life.

Over the next few weeks, he managed, on occasion, to cycle to the shops two streets away, by himself. Now and again I took him along the Moor path and held the seat. The prospect of one day joining me on a cycle run was daily held before him. Another new world? It re-vitalised his hope.

All this aside, there was a change in him, as a person, that was becoming more apparent as each day passed. The mischief had gone; the silly giggle and the jocular prank. Mingled with his periodic depression, this seemed a part of it, until I realised what was happening. He was growing up. He was rejecting his own childish ways. More and more, being with him was less like supervising a boy and increasingly like sharing with an adult. We never had to consult each other about what he wanted. We knew each other perfectly. This was not misery, but maturity. He was becoming companion to me, and he was not dull company.

Always, he had been an avid reader, preferably of holiday and school adventure stories. One intellectual lady had once reproached me, at the onset of his handicap, for letting him read Enid Blyton. But that relaxation and projection by imagination was just what he needed; easy, simple, fast-moving, satisfying stories about children; children who could run and climb and do all the things he couldn't do. His mind was so easily tired by classics that he had to strain to understand.

Then his taste, too, began to change and expand. He asked me about the heroes, throughout the Church's history, we regarded as saints. He wanted to know about the children who had seen apparitions of the Blessed Virgin, and talked to her, in Lourdes, Fatima, La Salette, Garabandal. He sucked in the information like a dry sponge. He was developing a thirst for the spiritual.

I was repeatedly surprised and shaken by his secret activities, unnatural in a boy typically scathing of piety. I'd go in one day and find him reading a book of prayers, written for adults, to Christ the Redeemer. I'd lift him up and a rosary would fall out from his clothes. There was one day, at Mass, he sat beside me at the end of the pew in his wheelchair, and I thought he was having a little doze. He had every reason to be tired. There were a lot of people and Communion was taking a long time. I teased him about it on the way home and he said unemotionally, unpretentiously, in a way that shamed me to the bone, 'I wasn't asleep. I was praying. For you.'

He couldn't walk to the altar rail, now, for his own Communion. I had to push him in the chair. One day, as we turned away from the rail and moved past the Lady Altar back to the seat he said, 'Stop. Leave me here with Her. You go.'

It was a dismissal I understood. How often had I not wanted to be alone, in my devotion? But it struck me hard that he was no longer a baby, nor yet a child. He was independent of me, in that respect; an individual under God.

I left him there, each time after that. It became a habit. He was out of my hands. Hadn't I given him to God, that day of his anointing, to take or to leave, to use as He pleased? All I willed, and for which I prayed, was the strength to live it, 'Just for today.'

CHAPTER 16

Up and down

The time had now obviously come for Martin to have a bed downstairs. To cut him off from the family circle was harsh cruelty, and this way, he could sleep any time. He didn't like the idea, and rebelled against the use of it, but those two flights of stairs had utterly defeated me. I couldn't carry him, and nor could I be running up and down on days when he was bedfast for hours. He wouldn't spend the night downstairs, and I had to sleep near him, so there was still one terrible journey each way, each day, when lifting him strained my own spine, and the only alternative was for him to crawl up, painfully, like a cat.

I couldn't leave him alone for long now. He lost his balance easily, and couldn't walk unless I supported him from behind, under his armpits. We were feeling morose again when a young priest, son of a neighbour we knew, came home on holiday from Rome. He was helping out in the parish, but not responsible for it, so had more freedom than the others. Martin had said drily one day, when movement was difficult, why couldn't we have Mass in *our* house for a change, instead of having to go to God's house all the time.

He was nearer the bullseye than he knew. House Masses were coming back, and it was possible for our young friend to say one privately, for Martin. The top of the bar was idea for the purpose, we couldn't afford alcohol and had the thing full of books. It was a Feast Day, and we gathered with us a group of friends who had come very close during the crises. Martin was both pleased and unaffectedly, justifiably proud, to have the familiar ceremony in his own living-room. Minds shuttled back to early Christian days, before churches, when all Masses were like this. There was a family warmth and a firm sense of community that endeared us to the idea.

After Communion, Martin played his record from Lourds, and some children's gospel songs. Everybody had a card from him, and he had them all sign the visitor's book. It was a tremendous boost for both of us, and we needed it. Just that morning I had discovered that his back was scorched by the heat treatment, and the skin broken. It wasn't the usual burn; his bottle was always well covered. This was due to sluggish circulation and an abnormal build-up of heat in the tissues.

It created a real problem though. The surface was raw and tender; it would have to be dressed. The heat of the bottle, which he wouldn't part with, was going to dry out the dressing very quickly and make it difficult to remove. The alternative was to deprive him altogether of the comforting heat.

Over the next few days, I tried everything; the exudate from the skin was foul, and many products made the skin bleed, it was so highly sensitive. Such unhealthy tissue heals very slowly, and I could see this dragging on for ever. Even without the hot water bottle, the dressings dried, and I had to hump him into a bath to soak them off.

Then I remembered a healing antiseptic that would not harden. Honey. We both ate it, but had never used it this way before and Martin reacted as though I was using marmalade. But it worked. Well-padded, it kept him comfortable. It picked off easily. When he was lying doing nothing, I took off the dressing to let the skin dry out. In a short time it was clean and healed.

The unpredictability of activity continued. One day he was incapable of anything but lying or sitting about, watching what I was doing. Then he'd get a sudden idea, and want to go out. It was stop everything, get him dressed and go, which was becoming increasingly difficult. From the waist down, he was getting larger by the day, his flesh swelling with fluid, as in heart failure, due to pressure on his main arteries. His feet were so bulky he couldn't wear shoes; it had to be slippers. He couldn't stand, so I had to lift him, then swivel him around into the chair, catching him as he fell. There was the cushion and blanket to arrange, the bottle to put in place, his tablets to beat back the pain, then the wheels to manoeuvre over the step. It was a tedious undertaking.

So more and more we tried to bring life into the house, to reduce his going out. I was busy with some preparation for television programmes, that involved talking to religious people about their work. When I explained how tied I was, these people always insisted on coming to me, instead of my going to them. There were also our own priests, from two parishes, and the men caught up in my writing, or Lay Apostolate. There were so many clergymen coming and going we had a notice made for the door; 'Beware of the Dog-collars'. Martin loved it. He thrilled to their male voices and the religious talk, and forgot his trouble for a while.

One man who did Martin a power of good was Bishop Anthony Galvin, the man who just a few months before hit the world headlines by saving Pope Paul VI from assassination. Martin was unmoved by headlines; he never saw them, but he very much wanted to meet a Bishop. He knew the day I was recording the interview. He could no longer accompany me to the studio and he missed it sorely, but the Bishop was such an amiable man, and so friendly with everyone, I told him about Martin. Immediately, he asked to be taken to see him, and duly arrived at the house. A generous man; a man of the people, who knew about suffering, poverty and hardship. A man with a big, loving heart and a kind of wisdom. He made Martin laugh, and gave him his blessing, his eyes soft compassion. After he'd gone, Martin sighed and said practically, 'Now I'm *sure* to get better.'

Out of the visitation came another blessing, as one good thing leads to another. A man who had accompanied the Bishop rang a few days later suggesting that, if

Martin were up to it, he'd come and take us out somewhere in the car. Martin was delirious with excitement. He loved cars, and hadn't been anywhere for such a long time. He wanted to go to the coast, to the fairground and amusement arcades. We could fold the chair and take it with us.

So one sunny morning the three of us fulfilled his dream. He played Bingo, winning me some cheap china and a strap of horse-brasses. He ate a man-size lunch in a restaurant, disposed of ice-cream and candy-floss, then had a ride on a roundabout that was way too high for me. I'll never foreget his radiant face, lit with delight, his frail and vulnerable little body, as he clung hard to the man's patient strength and swung up in the air. He wasn't a bit nervous. He came back and slept all night, the first time for weeks.

It wasn't to last. Inevitably the pain caught up with us. I made no appointment for anything public because I never knew whether I'd be able to make it. On one occasion though, I had been asked, months before, to judge a fancy dress competition at a garden party. Martin enjoyed such things and his topical, quick, spry wit usually gave me a good opening line. When this particular day came in sight, I informed them of my problem, and they insisted on sending a car. Once again he could be lifted out and do what was possible from the wheelchair.

But it wasn't to be. After only half an hour in the grounds, he was gripped by a spasm, rigid from his feet up, perspiring and unable to move his neck. We had to bring him home. As he lay on the bed, dejected and pale, I was arranging in vases the flowers I had been given, and he said cryptically, 'You'd better keep those for my grave.'

It was the very first time he had ever referred to death, and it went through me like a blade.

He had the air of, not a disappointed child, but a weary old man, utterly defeated by life.

'Nonsense,' I told him flatly. 'They'll be dead long before you are. Besides, the

Hoppings are coming.'

That gave him something to think about. Every year, we had a fairground of our own, just 200 yards from the house. It lasted a week, and had the proportions of a city festival. Last year he had gone with the children from the Home. This year we wanted to make it together.

One reason I hadn't dared tell him was that I hadn't any money. Sideshows, and rides and stalls come expensive. If he went, the others would have to go too. I couldn't do it, but I was committed now. Without fretting, I prayed.

That week, Martin was very low. School holidays were on us. I was overworked, overwrought and had less freedom to share with him. One morning in town, I called into a religious shop that I had once used as a poste restante in the days when I had no address. Martin had often run in there for me, picking up my mail, making the woman laugh with his funny ways. I hadn't been in for weeks, and they must be wondering how he was. So I made the effort, and was rewarded with the answer to prayer. As I left, one woman who had a fondness for both of us, and had given me faith many a time, pressed a note into my hand 'Get Martin something he wants,' she said.

That afternoon, two young teachers came, one of whom had taught Martin before we moved. They brought a huge basket of fruit, and letters from the children he once knew. He was dismally unresponsive. He seemed a little unwilling for them to see him as he was, or maybe he was remembering when he could go to school. But failure as a visit often seems, there is an underlying stimulus. An hour after the visitors had gone, Martin struggled up and said, 'Mam, let's go to the fair.'

I had to think quickly. It was a fine night. Now we had the money. I rang the taxi driver, and this time I could pay. He came, and in we piled, all five. He wouldn't leave us until he had Martin comfortable, with two hot-water bottles, three cushions, four codein and a blanket.

His striped hat, in the right colours, was stuck at a cheeky angle on his head. *He* wasn't going to be beaten by any old tumour, not with a hurdy-gurdy on the Moor.

As we went in the gate, the music hit his ears and he laughed, 'Listen, that's my record.' It was Al Jolson. I'd bought him the L.P. after we'd seen 'The Jolson Story' on television. No roundabout for him this time; there was nobody to lift him, but plenty else to be done. He played Bingo and won a fur doll. He rolled pennies, and knocked down tins. He posed and had his picture taken with a monkey, which promptly nipped his finger and ran off with his brother's cornet. It was a magical evening. Coming up the road home, clutching his treasure and winnings, and eating a bag of chips, he said, 'Thanks Mam. That was great.'

Unpredictability was evident in every day, also the response to a spur. One Sunday morning we didn't go to Mass. I'd been up all night. I was weepy for the want of help and relief. He was sombrely aware it was all his fault, which wasn't true. I had other stresses. We'd had to call the doctor to his swelling abdomen, and that depressed us both. He felt like a patient again. I felt a failure. How long could this go on, clutching at each day for a change, like the dead touching a radiator?

Came evening, and I suddenly decided I *was* going to Mass. I jolly well would not be beaten. Where was the point of it all, if I gave in now? So I poked my head round the door to tell Martin, who was watching television from his bed.

I was just moving out again when he yelled, 'Hey wait! I'm coming too.'

Oh no. All that paraphernalia. We'd never make it. I was so looking forward to just one hour of peace and solitude. But I couldn't deny him. We hurried. I had to run. But we made it, in time for Communion. Afterwards there was a little resurrection of something inside me. We went to the Ever-open store and had an ice-cream. He took an age selecting sweets for his tin; he never spent much;

it was variety that appealed. I pushed him back leisurely, enjoying the air. We ended the day happily, watching another film on television.

The spirit of pilgrimage eased much of our attendant frustration and recurring sense of helplessness. In our parish was an ancient shrine to Our Lady of Jesmond, long since a ruin and the property of the Corporation. Centuries before, it had been the magnet of pilgrims and the scene of miracles. The devout still went, privately. Each year came a procession, from the diocese. We were fortunate enough to have easy access to it, and to the well, defaced during the Reformation. Often we made secret journeys to that spot. It was the same lady as in Lourdes; a woman who could change the course of history.

One day I took Martin to the well, in search of the will to persevere. Such a visit never failed to result in something, however light or slight, to make life easier. I left him at the top of the steps, and went down with a jug. I came up and removed the blanket, to pour cold water over his aching feet. 'This is like the Last Supper,' I quipped.

He didn't comment. He simply pulled up his loose trouser legs and said significantly, 'Put some on my knees.'

His knees. He hadn't said anything about his knees hurting him. Willingly I bathed them, wincing inside me at the huge swelling, the tight skin and plummy oedema. Was this the child I had so recently scolded for screaming?

The track back was rough, with stones that must have jerked and jarred all his bones. All he said was 'Get moving. Get it over.' He never complained. It was a hot day, and a long push back, so I paused at our parish church for a breather. I parked the chair outside and told him flatly, 'One day, I'm going to write a book.'

'Oh yes,' he responded. 'Write about me.'

I looked at him, as I went inside, my cross and my glory, my joy and my pain.

And I promised him, 'Yes. I'll write about you.'

It was Her idea really.

CHAPTER 17

Put the light on Mam

During the second week of August, Martin complained of toothache, on the right, unaffected side of his face. It was understandable. No dental check-up had been possible since we'd moved. But when I came to actually examine the molar, and the area, there were other indications that made my mind lurch. His right eye-lid was swollen and pulled down unnaturally. There was a hard lump under his right jaw-bone. Sure enough, there was the same evidence of secondaries that I had first observed on the left side, five months before.

When I'd steadied, I smiled, gave him a drink and said brightly, 'Nothing to worry about. It wasn't. Within a few weeks the tooth would be pushed out by the growth.

I notified the Infirmary. I thought the specialist would be interested. We had been back to the clinic, just to let him examine Martin, but had politely refused a few days inside for radium to Martin's spine. I have given the child my promise and wasn't going back on it. I also knew what radium to a nerve centre could do. His leg and spine spasms had gone by now, and so had the acute pains.

Around this time there was something more to accept; he was having difficulty in reading. It took him a lot longer to get through a book, and when I asked why, he said the words were blurred. He had to hold the book very close to his eyes. One afternoon I brought in his new comics, to find that he hadn't read the previous ones. They were lying untouched by his bed. I didn't say anything. He behaved as he felt, and I didn't query anything unless it was harmful. I didn't buy any more.

Tiredness and discomfort were taking both his appetitie and mine. He couldn't lie down now, and had constant difficulty in finding a comfortable way to sit. This took a lot of fun out of the wheelchair rides and discouraged us both. Nerve-ends split without nature's healing balm of sleep; and to my dismay I began to snap at him.

He had a bell; shining, brass souvenir of a sea-voyage, given to him by a friend who thought it would help. It did too; a novelty but immensely practical. It saved him shouting, and also my asking if he needed anything. I had never resented it. But now the very ding of it began to tear my mind. A summons. Something else to do. One day, he rang it when I was fraught and having to drop everything to settle a noisy dispute between his younger brothers. On a reflex, I turned and yelled 'Oh, shut up Martin. SHUT UP!' It wasn't his fault. It was the gravest injustice. He never had taken advantage of me in that respect. But every woman has her limit and I'd been living at mine for months.

I put it right, but I mourned, and

feared that something insidious was creeping into our relationship. We'd always been so calm and unified. No matter what. It was Martin and me together, as one. There-in lay our strength. Now here was life dividing us. It was me against him. He sensed it too, and was worried, his little face falling into a sad frown, thoughtfully hesitant about ringing the bell again. He once said I never shouted like other mothers. I'd failed him. This wasn't me.

His back had broken down again into bleeding sores, from his shoulders to his seat. The pressure under his diaphragm was making him breathless as a pregnant woman. I couldn't be sure there was no disease around his throat and lived in dread of his one day choking to death.

In complete contradiction to all this, his mind and spirit were very much alive and alert, enthusiastic for movement and eager to throw off any impediment. He tried so hard to help, especially during the night. He *wanted* to recover, and he wanted so much to make life easier for me. He fought and fought the depressive pressure of symptoms that were mechanical in the main.

One day I knelt in church, the medical picture slipping like film through my imagination. Why couldn't somebody kill that tumour? It had a neck, that could be wrung; a root that could be destroyed. It could be cauterised. Then it would die, and be assimilated naturally. It couldn't eat my boy then, stealing all the nourishment his fighting system needed.

It would take a clever surgeon; an experimental one maybe, but they did it with brain tumours. In this case it would be crude and uncomfortable, but it could be effective. I was willing to take the risk, if it would give him a chance. I wrote to the pediatrician that afternoon; a mad leap in the dark. I also told him I was at the end of my resources and had to admit defeat as far as nursing was concerned. The other children must not suffer, and there just wasn't enough of me to go round. I had to have a break.

Telling Martin was something I delayed

until we had seen the specialist again. Meantime we lived by the minute, just hanging on, to God and each other. Impatient of anything that kept me from him, I felt all the forces of life conspiring to take him away from me. I wanted nothing so much as to leave all else to somebody else and just concentrate on him, but it wasn't possible.

One afternoon I took him along to church as usual, and we sat in the cool shade; candles flickering at Mary's feet. I'd pushed him, as I often did, to the front, and left him there, before the Sanctuary, whilst I went to look at the books. As I went back to fetch him, he turned, and with such a look of adult wisdom said seriously 'I'm not finished.' There was something imperious about his tone; almost as though *he* were the parent and I the junior. I retreated carefully.

From the aisle, I watched his face. He was holding a silent conversation with the source of all our guidance. All of a sudden, his face lit, he seemed to nod a little, then smile. He was smiling, as though opening some mystery that was closed before. He understood. In a minute or so, he turned, his usual self, and said 'You can come now.'

He told me nothing. I didn't ask. I left it between him and God. But when I broke it to him, that he had to go back into hospital, he took it like a man. He accepted, and he promised to do everything the doctors told him, and he trusted me that it wouldn't be for long. It wasn't easy, but he did it.

There was no possibility of surgery, or of treatment to his face. I still wouldn't let them touch his spine. But they could perhaps drain some of the fluid from his abdomen, relieving the pressure and tension, leaving him not quite so heavy to lift. Meantime, I'd be able to relax, as far as a mother alone ever can, and enjoy the bliss of sleep, knowing he was safe in other hands.

Just one thing he asked, before he went in. He wanted to be anointed. I knew what was in his mind. It had saved him before. I explained to him that this situation wasn't quite so critical; we did have the doctors and the hospital. The arrangement was made. But I knew how he felt, and I winced at parting too. We needed encouragement.

The night before he was admitted, I was putting him into bed in the attic when he said 'Put the light on Mam. It's dark.'

I was folding his clothes and looked, amazed. The night was light, and its sun streaming in through the windows. The impact of his confusion made my spirit sink, but I said calmly, 'Hardly worth it. You'll be asleep in a minute.' He was too. Ironically, he slept that night. But my heart lay awake late and wept.

Next morning I woke about five, to that same sun illuminating our impending separation. I felt it, more than I dared to think, but I did need relief. He'd be better when he came out. On that I hooked my mind and resolved not to grieve. We had mice in the attic. I could hear their lively scampering under the boards; now and then a squeak. I glanced across at Martin anxiously afraid they should waken him.

But he was already awake, lying there, not making a sound, just open-eyed. Thinking his bottle must be cold I asked 'What's the matter love?'

'Nothing,' he said with such a sad expression, 'I'm just enjoying being at home.'

The draining of his abdomen was no use. It wasn't fluid in there but the solid tumour. He was in a room by himself, and very ratty when I went in. 'Take me home. Please,' he pleaded. 'Take me home. It's awful in here.'

I argued and was stern with him, but he was a different boy. Gone was the gentle placid acceptance, gone was his security. Sobbing, holding onto me like a vice he whimpered and confessed, 'When I wake up and you're not there, I'm frightened.'

It was no relief to me either, his being away. I couldn't sleep. My body and mind were all geared to him. Nobody else knew his needs. Away from him, I was like a woman in love. I couldn't settle.

The strain was even worse. Visiting was virtually impossible, with the others to supervise and feed, but essential to us both. I had to let them all fend for themselves with cold meals, while I sat with Martin. On Sunday afternoon we watched the movie on television, while a lamp dried out the weals on his back. It was a portable set, at the end of the bed, and Martin couldn't see it. Another nail was crucifying his nature. The specialist had insisted he get rid of that hot water bottle. He was now on drugs instead and utterly miserable. He'd writhed and cried and yelled at first, in animal protest at being parted from his only comfort. But I backed up the doctor and explained he was inflicting these burns on himself. He couldn't come home until he had done as he was told. So he was trying.

Monday I went back to him again, not having slept above an hour. How could I, with him suffering so? The smile and the fight were gone out of him. He was passive and disinterested. His apathy was all wrong to me. His mind was sluggish and his spirit sublimated. He wasn't responding or communicating, except to limply hold my hand. He wasn't enjoying life the way he did at home. He'd given in.

I left him, with a struggle, and cried all the way back to the others. Was this the way I was to remember him?

It was Bank Holiday. I fed the children, then sat down with them an hour. They laughed and squabbled, and played. My eyes moved from them to Martin's empty bed. This was what he needed. Love, life and stimulus, not sedation and defeat. They didn't have time in there, to treat his mind with talking and take him out in the fresh air. In an institution he could only sink into stupor and despair. I jumped up.

I rang the taxi, and within an hour, I had Martin home; pale, muffled and swathed, but smiling, for the first time in days. He had developed diarrhoea, was flaccid with drugs and had his very first bedsore. But his burns were healed again, and he was detached from the cause. As

I rolled him back into his own bed he sighed and said, 'That's good. Now send for the priest.'

God was his anchor, and mine. I couldn't keep up his routine as before, but I could do something to lighten it. I told our young priest friend, now home again from Rome, about Martin's dependence on Communion, and he agreed to call each morning at the house, on his way back from church. We had the plasterer in, doing some very necessary repairs. One of them whenever he was there, made a point of carrying Martin for me, down to his wheelchair. He then agreed to come back and do something about the kitchen, which meant I wasn't going to be entirely alone. A cousin and a neighbour volunteered to help. It seemed, after all, we could manage.

Once the plastering was done, I could move Martin down on to the next floor, near a big wide window with a lovely view. I moved in beside him, and a new chapter began. It was to be one of the happiest and yet the heaviest of them all.

His sight continued to give trouble, and affect his few simple pleasures. Time and again I caught him using a torch, in broad daylight, to find the switch on his radio, or to wind his watch. One afternoon I found him listening to television with no picture to be seen. Moving to right the set, I made some remark, and he said practically, 'It doesn't matter. It won't make any difference. I can't see.'

Martin was completely blind.

CHAPTER 18

The summit

The bliss of those late summer mornings is indelible on memory. We woke early, and Martin switched on his radio. Instantly the room was filled with swinging youth, juvenile fun, the joy of living and the urge to get-up-and-go.

'Do you want your coffee now, love,' I'd ask, and he'd say, 'Yes please.'

Around his bed there was a peace and a lightness I found magnetic. It infused me with energy far more than the coffee could. The coffee was good though; decaffeinated, or dandelion, laced with honey and a pollen that gave us protein. We sipped, and talked, and planned what to do with the day.

On his dressing-table were letters, cards, holy pictures from all over the world. Every day brought another batch. All wanting Martin's prayers, all bringing us spiritual support that kept us up on a cushion of air. His signs and symptoms were still there, but they were beneath us. We had a world of our own.

He was surprisingly free of pain, and had been for some time. It was mechanical discomfort he suffered from; everywhere he sat, the fluid in his tissues drained to that spot, like sand in a bag, and he had to move. Since he couldn't move himself, it meant constant attention and assistance from somebody who could.

The doctor was calling daily now and we tried all ways to get rid of the fluid. Sometimes it worked. We also tried a new sleeping pill which Martin said made him feel 'like a fairy.' He woke a few hours later having been completely free of his cross and said, 'I'm having that *every* night.' But next day his mind was tired. We couldn't get the routine started. He needed constant stimulus, and was a drag for me. By the third night, the pill was less effective. He woke after two hours.

After a week, it didn't work at all. So I gave him a potassium tablet that looked the same, and returned to the old round. He slept for a short spasm, and woke immediately, always with that same, beautiful smile and, 'Yes please,' to all I suggested.

'I wish I could go to the big shops,' he asked me one day. 'Can't we get the taxi?' He was remembering the fair, and what he once could do. But that had been weeks ago. Even had we got the wheelchair into town, we'd never have got it around the store. He couldn't sit still in it above an hour, and I certainly wasn't up to the effort. I said we'd try, and then assisted him to forget.

His mouth was bleeding slightly, where the cancer had reached his tonsils and was invading his throat. The flesh on his monstrous legs was weeping night and day, through thick bandages. The skin was bruised and breaking down into ulcers. All his afflictions he took with quiet resignation, trusting me implicitly. Just once he said, as I pushed the wheelchair over the step into the street he could not see, 'Mam, when will I get my sight back?'

'When everything else gets better,' I assured him, 'that will too.' We still believed very firmly in miracles.

Because of this, I had to be very careful who I left with him, on the rare occasions when I was out alone. His faith was essential and must not be shaken. Had anything given him reason to doubt either God or me, the whole basis of his existence could have been fractured, and his security gone. I shared him only with those who believed in God and were loyal to me, and who believed absolutely in what we were doing.

His personality had undergone a radical and irrevocable change. This was a boy I never knew; a man in fact, who had outgrown his childhood absolutely. His detachment was quite marvellous in one so young, and in one who had so clung to his interests and preferences. His puppets lay lifeless in their boxes. His recent joy, a beautiful plastic building kit from which he made fantastic working models, was idle under the heap of others. Even when he could see, he didn't grumble. He let each one pass, as it became necessary, and accepted the loss. He moved his mind onto something that he *could* do, and began to enjoy that. He didn't grieve over the unattainable.

I'd promised him I was going to take him away for a few days, when it could be arranged. Just the two of us together. We planned it endlessly. He saw happiness in just what we were doing on our own, mentally and spiritually.

His peace-loving nature, once taken for cowardice, now reigned supreme. If he heard the little ones battling he'd say, 'Oh don't. You mustn't. Please don't fight.' They didn't. If one of them was bothering me, he'd divert the nuisance with 'Here, get a sweet out of my tin and leave your Mam alone.' One day I was the one to say something irritable to Judy, the dog, and Martin reproached gently, 'Oh don't. It isn't her fault. She doesn't understand.'

His sense of justice was easily inflamed, and we all went to him for sympathy. One afternoon his older sister was left to make the tea, and the two youngsters refused to eat it. She came to Martin in tears of disappointment. 'Oh, just let them starve,' said Martin robustly, taking her part. 'They aren't worth it.' She did, and I reckon they learned a lesson.

This wisdom in him was astounding. A friend was watching the news on television one night, near his bed. Martin overheard the noise of riots and fighting in America, with familiar gunshots and cries of 'Freedom'. Quietly he commented, as if from the depth of a life's experience, 'What this world needs to learn is freedom from hate.'

The instinct to offer up his self-denial for the relief of others had now become a way of life. He was deeply concerned about countries where children were not allowed to go to church, and had no way of learning about God. But along with this serious intent, went his dry, rich humour, that shot his suffering with gold.

I came in one afternoon to find him exhausted after a particularly restless session. 'Thank God you're back,' he said cryptically, 'I've converted Red China while you've been out.' That same wit made him comment one evening, when a particular brand of dog food was blazoned in a television commercial. 'You'd better get some of that for me Mam. It prolongs active life!'

Nights were bad, and getting worse. I took to making coffee every couple of hours. Since we couldn't sleep, we might as well enjoy being awake. It was a dim weary trail down to the kitchen and back, till Martin, in his quick consideration said, 'Why don't you fill a flask, then we can just pour it when we want it?' He was so practical. Thus the night duty began. I gave up all hope of real sleep, and we just lived a different kind of day while the rest of the family had their night.

Always, he tried to organise things to help me. If he heard his sister out on the landing with a friend, he'd call them in. 'Mam's busy and I need a lift,' he'd tell them. 'you can be my nurses.' His imperious tone and autocratic motioning always reduced them to giggling, 'Now you get there, and you there, and when I tell you...HEAVE..' There would be a brushing skid as the weight of him was slid into a better position. 'There you are. Now you can go. And don't think you're going to get paid.'

His urge to go back to Lourdes was instinctive. He had started a new fund which stood at five pounds. Every penny that came near him went into that box. We were going to go back, and take the candle with us, and light it in thanksgiving. It was something to look forward to. His appetite was voracious; he enjoyed his food, and we'd found an effervescent Vitamin C flavoured with orange that kept his mouth fresh, as well as soothing the growth. Once again the back molar came out, 'Good,' he said, relieved. 'Now we don't have to go to the dentist.'

Prayer we resorted to, and leaned on for the very practical reason that it worked. The thought of him dying in a blue fit of strangulation by that throat closing was a nightmare to me. There was absolutely nothing I could do. So one day, when he looked at me, terrified and said 'Mam! I can't breathe!' I felt my utter dependence on Our Father to my bones. 'Here,' I said, calmly, for there were other children in the room. 'You say your Rosary. I'll go upstairs and ask God what to do.'

I ran up into the attic, and I prayed. 'Please God don't let him die this way. Send it away. PLEASE,' I said my Rosary, somewhat hysterically, for the will of God is demonstrated in events, and must be accepted. Once you've submitted the plea, and rested your case, you must take what he sends.

I came down, and Martin was quietly, happily watching television. 'It's gone,' he said, as I came in. 'It's all right I can breathe again.' It never came back. He never again knew what it was like to have to gasp for air to fill his lungs.

The family were his delight. Evenings they'd put on a pile of records and do all the modern things; jigging about and yelling till he told them all straight, 'You're maniacs,' and sent them out. Then he'd lie motionless and listen by himself. Music to keep his mind moving. Music to remind him, places we had been. Everywhere I went I brought him something back; something to think around.

The peace in his presence was not for me alone. Visitors began to notice it. They couldn't understand how a boy so afflicted could be so happy. They sat, and they found it infectious. Who wouldn't want to come again? One man who came to us, in deep trouble, asked to be left alone with Martin. He wanted to pray. Whether with him, or for him, I wasn't to know. But when that man came down, he had the look of a man with a burden eased. 'I held his hand,' he told me, disbelieving, 'and I knew such peace.'

He was a rare judge of character, this child, and saw through people immediately. He knew at once where there was pride, hyprocrisy, lies lack of charity, particularly unkindness. 'Don't let her in again,' he said once as a stranger left, 'She is selfish and only came to see what I look like.' Curiously, he was right.

As I saw through his eyes, so he had to see through mine. Everywhere I took him now I had to talk. He'd still make an effort to come out with me, to church or to anyone's home. The strong arms of the decorator made him feel secure, and kept life's door open for us. His heightened perception made him live every minute he was able, and throw off sorrow as soon as it was gone. One night I was pushing him round to Mass. It was dark and the sky like a great wild country of hill and cloud, in colours of breathtaking majesty. I described it, and told him, 'There's a star, just one star, shining like a silver sword.'

'Like a cross,' he said.

I felt uneasy. A cross. A sword. The symbol of separation. I resisted it defiantly. 'Christmas,' I insisted. 'There must have been one like that at Christmas, all the way to the stable. That star is a sign Martin. Freedom. We're going to be free of all this.'

His books no longer readable, I took to reading to him. It lifted his mind and kept him thinking, away from his infirmities. I chose those that filled his mind with faith, and victory, and miracles. Stories of people who surmounted impossible difficulties, who bravely fought the battle of life, and won. One day he asked me to read the life of John Vianney; the smiling saint we'd seen in Lourdes, whose name I had taken; the clumsy farm boy who deserted from the Napoleonic wars and could argue down the devil himself. As the story developed, Martin listened, eagerly absorbing every word. John's love for his mother, his family life, his earnest desire to be a priest. At each point, where I had to stop, he'd ask 'That's not all is it? The book isn't finished?'

The words went so deep, I could see his thin face light, alter and register at certain points. John had a terrible time with his Latin. Martin laughed out loud when the Grand Vicar sympathised, 'They tell me the devil speaks Latin beautifully.'

Then that fateful sermon, when poor John tried to impress and convert his tough parish, got up in the pulpit, and found every word had left his head. Martin chuckled. That had happened to me once, on television. His face was enthralled when I read the Saint's rule of life 'Do nothing that is not pleasing to God,' and then cleared at, 'Heaven is where one *sees* God, face to face. Think of that...'

I looked up, and felt unease again. Martin was thinking. He was also possessed of the notion of sacrifice; giving up everything for something you want very much; offering all you have to God, for something in exchange, something only He could give. Heaven cropped up again, in a story about John Bosco, the acrobat turned priest who took ruffian boys off the streets till he had 400 in all.

'I wonder who mended their socks?' I paused to comment.

'His mother of course,' said Martin. He was right, as the story went on to prove. That Saint was once called to a boy who was dying, and had something to confess. Don Bosco absolved him and then asked, 'Would you rather stay here on earth, or go to Paradise?' The boy had just had a dream of Heaven, and he said without hesitation, 'Oh, Paradise...' and he died.

At that I realised what I was doing, and looked up anxiously at Martin. He was lost to reality. His face was thoughtful and troubled. Then it was eased, but I was afraid. Did he prefer Heaven to me?

CHAPTER 19

Trapped

Toward the end of September, the cushion of grace lost its filling and down we went. I simply could not take the strain. Martin's illness had progressed to a point where it must result in some crisis I dared not contemplate, yet his mind was hypersensitive. I was under pressure on all sides. There was no moving for us, to left or right. Only up. We prayed. Freedom for him, from this dreadful condition that had his bright spirit in a prison. Freedom, for me, from this burden of love that could no longer give. There was nothing I could do for him.

I slept near him now, on a settee, about two feet away from his face. I could reach out and touch him, any time. I hadn't slept for so long I hardly knew what I was doing, night or day. Once he stated flatly, 'I dread the nights. I get bounced around.' It was true. I was so weak, and in pain myself from a strained spine, I could only move him awkwardly and ungently. I could have let somebody come, for one night, to let me sleep, but he was so distressed by strangers, and I remembered the nightmare he had of waking up to find me not there. I wouldn't have it happen. He was so dependent and he needed me.

One night he turned in the dark and said 'Come in beside me.' I knew what he wanted; the warmth and security of those baby days, with arms enclosing him. He remembered the comfort it gave. It was Heaven to a child. So I tried. I really tried. But it was impossible. There wasn't anywhere I could touch him that didn't hurt. There wasn't anywhere he dare get himself close to me. 'It's no use,' he said practically, at last. 'It isn't going to work. You'd better get out.'

I crawled back to the settee and stifled a scream in me. Not to be able to give him what he needed. I lay back and throbbed with fatigue, letting tears I thought silent go their way.

'Oh, don't cry,' he pleaded. 'Please don't cry.' He was so acutely sensitive to my suffering, he always knew.

The only real relief he had was when somebody sat and massaged his back, where the tumour was, relieving the pressure a little from the outside. If he could listen to a story at the same time, it helped. He enjoyed being cleaned and changed; I never made it a compulsory routine. I waited until he asked. 'I'd like to be washed now.' Then I bathed his little face, almost transparent in emaciation, and cleaned his mouth, and brushed his teeth. Smoothing the soft sponge across the blue-veined skin, I felt not a flicker of resistance. He was so patient under it all. I remembered the squirming, rebellious school-boy who couldn't keep still, who reluctantly offered his soap-and-water martyrdom for the holy souls. Was it only three years ago?

We put all sort of things into the water

now, to make it pleasant for him. It had become a holy ritual. Someone brought us water from Mount Carmel. Martin said the heat made it smell of oranges, and he 'felt good.' There was water, too, from the well at Jesmond, and the last of what we had from Lourdes. It soothed him, and satisfied me. I was *doing* something.

All life, as we knew it, seemed to be running down. The clock from Lourdes, defective from the start, had stopped and wouldn't go. Whenever I *had* to go out, which was as rarely as I could make it, he knew instinctively how I was going to feel, and made it easy for me. 'You go,' he'd say unselfishly. 'Don't worry about me.' But when I came back, his whole being leaped across the room and he gave a little gasp, 'At last!' It was an ordeal for him. His interest in life was waning rapidly. One day a friend helped get him in her car, and we went for a ride round; something he loved. I stopped at a Supermarket and came out excitedly at what I'd found. 'Look Martin. French bread.

Lourdes...remember?'

He looked, his eyes dull, and nodded, quite unmoved.

Another day, we'd been shopping with the chair. I heard the train. I ran, and missed it by a second. 'Oh dear,' as it disappeared. I was disappointed in myself, at having failed him again.

He shook his head. 'It doesn't matter.' Nothing mattered. He didn't want his records on. He didn't want any visitors. He didn't want the children in. He wasn't interested. Yet he, himself, didn't seem conscious at all of what was happening. Feeling him slipping away from me, I could hardly bear to be with him at all, yet as my grief possessed me, when I was behind him, pushing him, out of sight, he'd say with genuine curiosity, 'What are you crying for?' He wanted me, but he was detached from me, in a way I found crucifying.

During one very bad night, when the world seemed red and sore, I'd had such a struggle to get him on and off his bedpan. Weak and limp with exhaustion, I let out the worst thing I could possibly have said, 'Oh, it's no use Martin. I can't manage. You'll have to go back into hospital.'

His little face crumpled, troubled. He said nothing. But I could see thought digging deep in his honest soul. Later, utterly consumed by despair, I wept unashamedly. 'I don't believe in God anymore. There's no God!'

He didn't say anything, or move. It was like ripples against a rock, my losing faith. But later when I came in, he was sitting on the edge of the bed, his bony frame resting on his bulky middle, supported by those ghastly leaden limbs that seemed to grow into the floor. His little face was tilted up to the light, his sightless eyes roaming the ceiling as though looking for a peep-hole. As he heard me come in, without turning he said softly. 'You know Mam, I love you. I wouldn't do this to you if I could help it.' It broke me. He was so gentle, and there was nothing I could do.

Somehow it passed. We reached out

and clung to another day. October 3rd was the annual pilgrimage to Jesmond, and he wanted to go. We made plans, to get him there, then concentrated on the in-between. October 1st was a Friday. I was in church alone, pleading our case, and had such a sense of let-down. A disappointment. I knew not where, or to what it referred. I just knew myself prepared. We'd had so many. What was one more?

The next day, I took him to Mass in the morning at the church by his old school. Our young priest had gone back to Rome, and a parish can't cope with daily Communion for the sick. It was the only thing in life that gave us hope, so we made that if nothing else. He couldn't swallow it now, without a drink before and after. It was my habit to take a small screw top jar with me, but this day I'd forgotten. My memory wasn't what it was. I had to ask the priest's housekeeper for a drink, and she went to get him a glass.

After Mass, we did as we always did; walked slowly down the High Street, and

I described what was in the shop windows. He was interested, but not as he used to be. I came to a bakery and said, 'Oh Martin, there's a cake in the window just like yours. A football pitch.' He nodded, but said nothing. Birthday. Was it only a year ago? It was coming up again in two weeks time. What on earth could I get him? All his wants, in that sense, were gone.

It was a cold day, and his hands were blue. His poor circulation. Nylon mitts were no use. He had to have something warmer. I stopped and bought him a pair of fur ones. That delighted his heart. I'd never been able to afford them, and couldn't now, but I'd have robbed the bank nearby to see him comfortable. We reached the sweet shop, and he made his usual bossy selection to the delight of the assistant.

Next day, Sunday, the pilgrimage was all. He was ready two hours before the car was due, quite sure this was THE day. Never, ever, had we come to deadlock and not had it eased by this journey. Today was something special. Today we had a new hope.

We parked outside the Shrine. He couldn't get out. He couldn't sit for long either, and I had to support him from beind. My hands were firmly down behind him, keeping his spine from the pressure of the seat. Those who knew him came across and had a word. Some wept as they left, but he couldn't see. One friend ran out of the crowd with a package. Her daughter had been to Fatima, and brought back a picture for Martin, of the boy. Francisco, who was at the apparitions and had died soon afterwards. Martin held it tight in his hand.

The hymn rose

> 'Sojourners in this vale of tears,
> To thee blest advocate we cry.'

I whispered encouragingly to my baby. 'Hang on love. Mary will do something. She always does.'

The prayers rose; rhythmic, repetitive. And Martin confessed wearily. 'Mam, all I pray for is sleep.'

We came back with a sense of complete

anti-climax. It was over, and nothing happened. We'd clung to this day. I began to feel depressed.

But not Martin. He sat on the edge of his bed, his face all lit with a new fervour and said, 'Mam, I feel like eating a Christmas dinner.'

'You must be joking! In October?' Not only that, there was so much growth in his mouth, he'd have trouble getting anything down that was thicker than gravy. Then I had an inspiration. Something began to register. There was a shop open; always open. 'Wait a minute love. I'll get you your dinner.'

I dashed out, and came back with a dozen tins of strained baby foods; chicken, potato, gravy, pears, and ice-cream. He ate the lot. I spooned it in and he swallowed it so fast you'd think he hadn't eaten in a week. Then he sat back and licked his upper lip and said, 'Thanks Mam. That was GREAT,' and ordered, 'Get me some more in for tomorrow.'

I did. Then I got the others fed, and into bed. We were looking forward to the film on television. I'd seen it before and had told Martin about it. The nuns came to see him. After they'd gone, I washed him, and put his pyjamas on. He didn't seem very interested in the film after all, so I didn't bother. It was of no interest to me, without him. He seemed a lot more interested in sleep, so I made him as comfortable as I could, and then left him while I went to clear up.

When I was finished, I went to look at him. He was lying, completely relaxed, his face sideways on the pillow. A wisp of a smile wreathed his mouth. His eyes were closed. I kissed him and said, 'Goodnight my love.' His happy 'Hmm....' indicated that he'd heard.

There was no point in my staying up. The opportunity to rest was too good to waste. I rolled, just as I was, on to the settee near him, knowing full well I'd be disturbed again within the hour.

CHAPTER 20

Freedom

I woke to silence. I woke to a sensation that I had slept too long. It was daylight. Wondering, I struggled up, unaccustomed to this freshness in me. It was wrong. I must make Martin coffee, and get him washed.

I moved across to him. He hadn't moved. He was exactly as I had left him, to the lie of his head. But the smile was gone. The face was tense and stiff, the mouth fallen open. My hand reached out to feel him, icy cold. 'He's gone.' The fact of it escaped me emotionally, as my mind accepted the reality. God has acted. God has made His will manifest. We are relieved.

I must protect the other children. They mustn't see. This alien thing on the bed could only shock and frighten them; this hideous shell was not Martin. He was gone. He'd gone and hadn't stopped to say goodbye. He hadn't even woken me. Mary had given him sleep, and then her Son had taken him. Jesus had been. He'd take him by the hand I knew, and he would be willing. I just wish...no I didn't. I was glad, he hadn't told me. I couldn't ever have said goodbye, not to my Martin.

Pain shafted through me, but it didn't fell me. I was sustained. I persevered and made my mind concentrate on the living. But first I went into the next room, and sent up a searing prayer to a saint who had left me to live alone. He was all right. I knew he was. We had friends in high places. Smiling John Vianney and strong John Bosco. Francisco and Jacinta from Fatima. He was all right. He was happy, and free. He wasn't alone.

Friends. I had to tell them, all the peole who had prayed. Now they had to know, what God had decided. I needed them. I sped upstairs and typed a few notes, then cycled around to deliver them, Judy snapping gaily at my heels. Dogs have no idea. Suddenly it came to my mind. 'Be kind to Judy. She's only a dog. She doesn't understand.' I must be kind to Judy.

I wanted somebody to come. Somebody to break this awful silence. I got the other children out to school. I rang the doctor. He said it was merciful, and left me a couple of tablets to take at night. Then they came. They held me, and let me cry, and they took some of my pain. I was about hysterical, by then, with memories; his voice, his lovely smile. 'You know Mam, I love you...' and 'Don't cry. Please don't cry.' I tried to stop crying. I just talked, and talked, and talked. These didn't know, these good ones, what we'd lived, the past few weeks. They didn't know the hero he was. what he'd been through. They had no idea what God could do. They remembered a boy. I'd lost an adult. I'd lost Martin. He wouldn't let that sustencane fail. As it flagged, he raised it. I once picked up his exercise book. On the first page was a spelling test from school; all right as usual. The first word was 'believe'. The scond was 'hoping'. I must believe, hoping. His message to me.

The day was different, not like any other day, and yet it was the same. I had to take his coat to the cleaners, with the Lourdes badge on the sleeve. Back up the High Street where we'd just been. I had to take those tins back to the shop. Maybe they'd refund the money. No use to him now. Lourdes. I must go back. I must go and thank her. She knew what she was doing, that Mother of mine. She knew I couldn't have taken this in advance. She distracted me. I couldn't have lived, and looked after him, if I'd known he was going. I had to believe he wasn't. I had to *believe* it. Only she could make me believe. I couldn't have looked after him, had I really felt it was going to end this way. I couldn't have nursed him dying. He had to be living, healing, improving. There had to be health just around the corner. Something to keep me going, at full strength, my reach always exceeding my grasp. I couldn't have been what he needed otherwise. I had to believe, or I couldn't have made *him* believe. She was a wise Mother. And she knew me.

Just one more thing I did for his little body. I lifted his head and put it on a blue quilted pillow, one I had rarely used. It was blue as the sky; blue as Our Lady's mantle. Blue as his eyes. Not until it happened did death come on the scene, and he never knew it. He died looking forward to life, and moved on into ecstasy. Martin was free. Martin was out of that terrible cage. He could go anywhere. He could see the shops and ride the lift, and ring the bells and run away. He didn't need the wheelchair any more. He didn't need me.

That night, when they'd taken all that remained of him to a chapel of rest, I took the pillow. His little voice told me, 'Come beside me Mam. Come in beside me.' We could do it now. I climbed into his bed, and he was close to me; as close as he had been as a baby, in my arms. I let my head rest in the imprint where he had been and prayed, 'Martin baby, let me sleep. Don't you be the one to keep me awake.' I didn't need the tablets.

I knew what the day after death can be, and expected to be crucified, as reality hit consciousness. But I woke to baby kisses on my face, and the words, 'I love you.' It got me downstairs before I missed the radio. I must break the routine. Now. I must detach myself. No use looking for things to be the same. Must plan them differently, now. I'd been round to the church, an hour after I found him. I knew the only way to live with this was to deepen other relationships. I had to love other people, now, the way I'd loved him. I had to be the mother to the others, he had taught me to be. They had no fear or dread of death. They saw it as a doorway. No drawn curtains and red eyes for these children. Martin had Heaven. It was a joy. As I wrote to a friend, 'The tumour is dead. Martin lives. Is that bad news?'

Letters came pouring in, all congratulating. Me on my gallant lad, whose courage was an inspiration. Me on my achievement, with his co-operation, getting him up God's mountain. Congratulations. It was more like a wedding. On the step, a few hours after I knew, there was a spray of flowers for me. There was no name, just a message, 'For the mother of the child, from another mother.' They felt it for me.

The night sleeping, and the morning waking, kept me up till after the funeral. It was the Feast of Our Lady of the Rosary, and all was white and blue. I wouldn't have money spent on flowers, when there were children homeless and in need. It was directed to the Diocoesan Rescue Society. Just one cross of white from his school, was laid with him. Then at the last moment, just before I left, a relative sent a bouquet of beautiful pink roses. I took them to church and put them at Mary's feet. For Her, from him. It was Martin's doing.

The school had a service for him, in the morning, in the church where he made his last Communion. The children had composed their own prayers that moved me to the soul. They asked Martin's blessing on his class, and all the needs of that community. The priest paid public tribute to his faith, love of God and patience. His last journey in this life had been a pilgrimage, to the Mother of God. It was a moving testimony.

In the afternoon I attended the funeral in a scarlet blazer. I refused to be subdued. He loved life, and colour, and we had reason to be gay. God's healing is not ours. Martin was cured of his condition; the human condition. Now he could help, heal us. From the Blessed Sacrament came the throbbing assurance 'I love you' in the atmosphere to me; as of a spirit released. It didn't budge the basic rock of grief, but it did prevent me from foundering on it.

The girls from the Grange, and one of the Sisters, sang 'The Lord's my Shepherd' at Communion. Going to the rail myself, I kissed the name on the box; the last kiss I could give him here. Coming out I saw the taxi-driver, the decorator, the priests and the laity, all Martin's V.I.P's, who made life worth living for him. People who had helped. People who were still helping. Strong hands to hold.

They buried him across the road from the Children's Home that once took him in. I stood and listened, and it didn't move me to anything much, except in that it is always a moving experience. I was full of Martin's spirit. There was enough in me to burst. The idea of *him* imprisoned in that box was utterly ridiculous. They couldn't bury that imp. All the same, I took one rose, from those sent by the school, and I threw it in. A rose is truth, purity and beauty. We had all three. A perfect love. A dark night and a fountain of grace; the heritage of all who believe. I'd clung, in love, to his cross and his death of self. Now I had a glimpse of his glory, and his happiness. He was telling me.

God had put him into my arms nearly eleven years before, a puny, wailing thing. I loved him on sight. I loved him before he was born. I taught him all I knew. I taught him all God had taught me. What more can a mother do? I gave him back to God, when the time came, when my purpose was done. A child who offered his life, as he surely did, to see his mother relieved. As surely as any son who ever went to war, in defence of his home and family, that boy died for me; my little modern English martyr, a victim of the plague, who saw me suffering and had wanted to do something, and had nothing to offer but himself. A boy who would rather die than be taken from his home and family again.

So God took his sacrifice, and then detached him, and let his life run down. Now God had given him a life that would never end. No harm could come to him, ever again. No pain, no suffering, no separation, no death, no disease. He'd never again know cold, or ridicule, or fear, or black fatique, or loss or love as we who are left must know. Martin was safe, for all time. His last pilgrimage was done.

After the funeral, when I was alone, I went over his legacy to me. He'd left me his watch, with the blue dial. He'd left me £7.53p to go to Lourdes. He'd left me his smile, and his bright spirit, and the memory of his love. By then, the pin-prick of reality had punctured the air-cushion again. All I could feel was that he had left me. The dreaded separation had begun.

But among the treasures that remained of his short experience in this world, I found a page one day; just ripped out of a cheap note-book. In pencil, in very young print were the words, 'thank you for a lovely day in my life.' He was glad he was born, that child of mine. He was grateful for the experience. I hadn't failed. I hadn't lost him. It was my consolation that I had done all I could.

He was born to die, my baby. A boy who wouldn't fight, until he had to fight for life, then he never lost faith in victory. He was a hero in the battle of life. No matter what they say, we won.

He did all the will of God for him, and that is what he was born for.

CHAPTER 21

In retrospect

Death is a fact of life, and there is no reason why it should be easier for me than any other mother. Death is a supreme test of faith, and in a matter of two weeks after it hit me, I was left wide open to the devil of grief. Long, lonely nights weeping cut glass out of my system. Days when every sight and sound was a dagger in me. The throbbing nearness of the train put my brain through a bread-slicer.

The mother-child relationship is particularly vulnerable to separation and jealousy. The deeper the bond, the more difficult it is to get interested in any other. I was not only stricken but hurt, that after all we had been to each other, Martin should choose to be with anyone but me. Even God. Where could he ever be happier than we were together?

The bitterness of desolation in such a separation is always greater when a child has been completely dependent. He left me with an expanded heart that nobody else could fill. He came so close, we two were one. Nor had I realised how utterly drained I was, in myself, after such a strain. I didn't cancel any of my appointments. A week after his death I was out taking a meeting where nobody knew. But it couldn't last. I collapsed into a state of mental, emotional and physical exhaustion, with recovery a long way off. Bereavement is amputation without anaesthetic at the hands of a lunatic. Shock is inevitable, then the victim has to be treated as convalescent. There has to be a gradual adjustment according to the individual. A period of mourning is essential.

Martin was better off, I told myself, and this was my sacrifice for him. When a soul weeps, it doesn't make a noise, it bleeds. So the soft, self-wounded pelican bled. Gradually, as my strength returned, in very uneasy stages, I was able to follow the recipe for heartache; work, company, distraction, and just enough activity to make me tired enough to sleep at night. My natural eagerness for people and causes set me working for charities; all those connected with what we had suffered. Television was an indescribable ordeal. I'd drawn power for myself from his weakness and determination. His love had given me confidence. It was something we shared, and I had to go on alone. I stayed up to watch one programme, recorded when he was alive, and never did it again. I knew my limitation.

It was six months before I could go to the grave, and it broke me utterly. From then I found I could do it more frequently. It became a place of pilgrimage. It was a year before I really came up out of the depths and began to climb back to what was normal for me. Progress is slow, and by degrees, with frequent relapse, especially at emotive times like Christmas, at school events and on anniversaries. 'Let go the dead and hang on to the living' was my constant exercise. And eventually it worked. I deepened other relationships and let them take me over. I was trained to acceptance and experienced in resignation. I had the will to pull out of the pit.

Life went on, and the raw, gaping wound he left began to heal. The Corporation changed the lock on the gate to the well, and it was closed to me. The Ever-open store closed too, and was empty for a while. The new owner didn't know about Martin. I began to read John Vianney, John Bosco and Enid Blyton to Martin's brothers, whose reactions were entirely different. One, aged 8, inherited the bicycle, and within a few weeks it had been stolen.

The youngest, then six, took ill shortly after Martin's death. I pounced on the opportunity to be to him what I was to Martin and fill the hole in my soul. I tucked him on the settee, with Martin's pillow and Martin's toys, seeking solace for myself as much as the child. He eyed it all with mixed feeling, then said shrewdly, 'I'd better not go to sleep. I might go to Heaven.' And a few months after Martin, the priest who had arranged the funeral had followed him, also through cancer; the modern plague.

Only now, looking back and knowing the end of the story, can I see it all clearly, in the context of our environment. Faith is stronger for the testing, and as mine returned it reiterated all I had said and done. Faced with the same problem again, I'd do exactly the same; treat the patient as improving, give him everything conducive to sound health and strength. Use all natural resources and avoid anything chemical or artificial. Abandon the medical profession entirely, except for assistance with nursing, and free medicines. Use drugs only when necessary, and leave the rest to God.

Cancer is not infectious or contagious. There is no reason why it shouldn't be nursed satisfactorily at home. It is not incurable, and God is not bound by the laws of medicine, so the course is unpredictable. The switchback of hope and disappointment we endured is typical. One hour Martin was felled, out of action completely. The next he'd be outside wearing a wig, having a crazy photograph taken. One day a visitor would call and assume him at death's door. After she'd gone, we'd be streaking across the Moor in giggles to fetch iced lollies. To enable such a patient to get the absolute maximum out of life, there must be a minimum of regulation; a flexible routine. That is not possible in an institution.

I was fortunate in having a completely open mind on the matter of treatment. In my nursing days I had seen some disastrous failures, and cases that defied medical opinion. I was free of any professional prejudice, had no particular axe to grind, and wasn't worried about upsetting any academic apple-cart. I wasn't living in any 'thought climate' obstructive to free reasoning, and I wasn't learned enough to miss eternal truth. So I was as ready to listen to the osteopath and naturopath as to a radiologist. I found the first two more skilled in the relief of suffering, and I still believe that nutrition has a great part to play in the prevention, management and even cure of a malignant condition.

Martin was a poor example in this respect because his leg prevented him from taking plenty of free exercise. Then his sore mouth prevented the intake of bulky foods. His palate was used to the sweet and fizzy so beloved by children of this generation, and it was late in the day to make a change. The site of the tumour, causing impediment to nerve force and build-up of pressure and sluggish circulation, prevented the free elimination of toxins. But on days when his sytem was clear, he was so considerably improved in every respect of his condition, I could see the principle working. Bearing in mind how far the disease had advanced long before he died, he must have had a very strong constitution, and that was not so before his diagnosis. It can only be put down to his diet.

'Natural' remedies of any kind are

widely ridiculed and frowned on in our society, simply because they are not commercial. Our whole economy is based on buying and selling; profit and return. Nobody can make a quick fortune out of fresh air, exercise, breast-feeding and the rhythm method of birth control. So money is not put into research, and the methods are not given the big benefit of psychological, high-pressure advertising. They do not interest the mass media, so do not reach the bulk of the population. It is for a small hard-working, experienced minority to get the facts before an ignorant, apathetic nation, and they get little encouragement. Drugs are a money-making proposition, widely advertised. People have come to think they can't live without them. A fallacy many times repeated without contradiction earns acceptance by sheer volubility. Millions actually believe aspirin is good for them.

Why use a drug when there are natural antidotes? They are effective, virtually harmless, non-addictive, and there is no danger of overdose. Some are expensive, but they wouldn't be if they became more popular, and thereby a paying proposition. Some drugs are very effective in the short term. Others hold out hope of a cure. Radium is a valuable discovery, and surgery can relieve, but to say that radium, surgery and drugs are the *only* way of tackling the condition is recalcitrant in the extreme. Diet is important, and disease an ignorance of elementary rules. We must treat not only symtoms but causes. We must treat the whole person. And we must work on prevention. We must fight the systematic pollution of our basic necessities such as food and air. While man wilfully despises the contracted balance of nature, the Pied Piper of cancer is stealing away our nation's children in their sleep.

The two big fears associated with cancer are of death, and of pain. Nobody wants to either suffer or die. But facing the facts means being thrown back on to one's whole philosophy of living and one's resources of courage. If these are absent, or inadequate, then a major part of the torment in all concerned is going to be mental and emotional, aside from any disease. And mental stress has an effect on cancer. Martin did not begin to demonstrate symptoms of any kind until he sensed tension in the home, and he had to watch me suffering. When we were wrenched apart, his condition deteriorated rapidly. Suffering can be relieved in many ways. It varies according to the individual. Worry and boredom can cause physical pain. But one thing is sure. Fear will make it worse.

Medicine can do nothing to relieve the fear of death. Few on a medical staff are able to talk about it. Facing it is essentially a matter of belief plus experience. For us, our basic philosophy was rock, and able to take the shock. We knew fear, but we did not live in fear. We had somewhere to go. Only God knows when we shall die. If we co-operate in life, we shall be prepared, and trained to it.

To some I must have seemed a lunatic, with my fanatic faith in Martin's recovery that survived so many disappointments and did not accept death until it happened. But in face of such tragedy, one must either hope or despair. We chose to live in hope, which is the spur to endurance. When I think of all the people I have seen, in hospital and in their homes, or expensive private rooms, dying like animals with no faith, not a hope and nobody to love them; with nothing to look forward to but a black oblivion, I know I did the right thing. Too many cancer victims begin to die when they hear the diagnosis. They think of themselves as already dead. Treated along with others bearing the same tragic tag, they are surrounded by death, thinking death, propelled into death long before it is necessary, and often taking a long time to die. Hence the talk of 'human vegetables' indescribable agonies and euthanasia.

Martin didn't die until he was dead. Literally. His mind was keen and his senses normal until the end. It is my consolation that we never ceased to be able to communicate, and to enjoy life together. Our Christian child-like nature responded wholeheartedly to the mood of the moment, forgetting danger ahead or grief behind.

Should I have told him? I don't see why. He had nothing to gain by that foreknowledge. He was happier, till the end, looking forward to this life and a complete cure. He had no property to dispose of, no justice to see done, no confession to make to someone he had wronged. He was happy. He would have been troubled at the mere wisp of a suspicion of leaving me, even if death itself had not alarmed his natural mind. He knows now what I could never tell him, and is grateful I know.

What really angered me was the opinion of the ignorant that he would be better off dead. To attempt to explain death, and what lies beyond, to the living, is like trying to explain this life to the yet unborn. I knew there was only joy ahead for him, because his life was blameless. But I never for one second seriously entertained the idea that he should be hurtled into that eternity by my own design. Life is sacred, and entirely subject to the will of God, who alone is qualified to handle such awesome power. We interfere at our peril.

It is so unwise to judge by appearances, or even imagination. To outsiders, Martin must have looked grotesque and difficult. To me he was always beautiful. Not until his death, when there was only the physical body there, did I fell any aversion. I loved him. He didn't really begin to live until I knew he was going to die. He outlasted his medical verdict by several happy months, and his was a *useful* life. He loved me, and he made *me* happy, for a start. So with his family and friends. He brought out the best in people, as I very soon realised to my surprise, after he'd gone and some of them reverted to type. He moved the hard and cold heart to *feel* something, and this they then acted on toward others.

People were changed at the very sight of him. They went back to their own homes, their own lives and trials, with a gratitude and fervour they didn't have before. His courage and dry, dazzling humour were an inspiration to others with far less to complain about, and they imitated. They left him, and felt concerned about all suffering humanity and set on *doing* something about it, not letting it settle comfortably on the periphery of life. He was a challenge to conscience that many of the sophisticated badly needed.

He had a function in life, my precious invalid. He pointed out what a mess this clever generation has made with the scientific and chemical forces at its disposal. He illustrated the utter failure to solve everything from a bottle, or with a machine. He demonstrated our dependence on divine wisdom. He reminded that life is unpredictable, and tragedy ever near. He kept people in touch with reality. He was, himself, incapable of evil. He showed how happy are the good. He appealed to what is finest in human nature, and brought it whizzing to the surface. He inspired compassion, honesty and humanity. He gave and he responded to love. He generated love.

For that reason I took on the current moves to have euthanasia legalised, with a mixture of disgust and horror. What right have so many people to talk so much about a situation they have never seen, let alone lived? They imagine how they would feel, and shout to have it put into Law. They fall for a theory, an argument, an abstract idea. They act on their own intrinsic fear. They discuss death in cold blood, without reasoning, research, or recourse to the people involved. They exercise organised pressure on the mass media, giving their ideas power and push on vulnerable minds that passively accept it as original and true.

They set aside the fact that we are all human, and will react to the circumstances according to certain norms of behaviour typical of man since man began. Death as an escape from life is nothing new. It is pagan, backward and decadent.

I saw euthanasia, twenty years ago, when learning about nursing. It was abhorrent to me then, and is now even more so. There is enough, without giving it free rein and the blessing of the State, which millions now look on as God. Present medical practice leaves plenty of scope for mercy. Few medical men will watch suffering and not move to relieve it. Legislation would put power into the hands of the unscrupulous, who have no conscience, and no respect for the human person.

I'm not afraid of suffering, or death. I am afraid of people who think they have the right to decide who should live and who should die. I do not trust those who airily claim to know who is useless, or even who *wants* to die. Emotional, spiritual and mental pain can be worse than physical ravages. Don't we all, at some time in life, want to end it?'

Of course there were days I wished Martin out of this life. There must have been times he wished it himself. But they passed. To have used any one of them as our overall verdict on life would have been ludicrous. Those days it wasn't the cancer to blame, but financial, social and domestic pressure which could, and ought to have been relieved. Martin lived through his darkest hour. God took his pain. Had I, during the worst moments, consented to euthanasia, I'd have missed the climax of his life; his greatest achievement and the source of my consolation now.

What euthanasia really means is, death to the unloved and unwanted: those whom society rejects as being imperfect, or serving no useful purpose. Pressure of publicity in this respect has the diabolical effect of making people *feel* unloved, imperfect, useless and unwanted. By even discussing the proposition, we are creating more suffering for them and sapping their will to live. Martin was undignified, but he was not conscious of it until some insensitive person forced him to feel it. The cancer did not make him suffer nearly as much as did the callous inhumanity of our public services, and the cruelty of individuals. Overall, throughout his ordeal, I suffered far more than he did. Would anyone have suggested mercy-killing *me?* To push euthanasia on grounds of relieving suffering is a specious deceit. Anyone who really loves humanity wants all people to enjoy life; the weak, while they live, to be protected, relaxed, happy and cared for. I'll wage war on any government that calls itself civilised and offers murder as the solution to cancer.

I have worked for years among the suffering, and disabled, the mentally and physically handicapped. I never yet met one who expressed the wish to die. They are among the most cheerful, determined, courageous and active people. I have ever known. Not one person involved in caring for them, takes the theory of mercy-killing seriously. It is irrelevant. If anyone does want to die, it is because, in some aspect of life, society has failed where there is a dire need. We should be aiming at changing society, not killing its victims. But it is so much easier and cheaper to kill people than to make their lives worth living.

Pressure groups talk as though death were the end of the problem. The ultimate relief; the final curtain. They assume there is no consciousness after death, and are gravely unaffected by the reaction of those who are left, for whom this life goes on. The impact of death is no minor thing, and rarely transient. It has to be experienced to be appreciated. I would rather die myself, than have to live and feel responsible for the death of another. I have seen relatives say 'yes' at the time, and regret it for the rest of their lives.

Death is a decision that cannot be revoked. There is no going back, undoing what has been done. That anyone ill in this country should *prefer* to die, is surely an indictment on us as a nation; our concern, our compassion, our government and our health services. There is plenty of money going on other things.

People in the circumstances I had to live, are just not in a state to be making rational life-or-death decisions. They are open, vulnerable, dependent; looking for a lead. They will fall readily for any idea put into their minds to relieve the sheer anguish, especially if that idea comes from someone in authority. They are not really choosing freely, but submitting to something they cannot fight, just as many women and young girls submit to an abortion they are secretly against.

There is, deep-seated in all of us, an instinct toward the inviolability of human life. Sublimated by pressure for a time, it will nevertheless survive and rise. Then the consequences of our actions will be seen in sharp relief, indelibly marked on the mind. Such guilt is very difficult to remove. I loved my child, and in my love I would have done anything to relieve him. But I now know, with the experience of his death behind me, and yet still ever with me, that had I for one moment ceased to fight to feed his life and give it quality; had I, at any time done anything to hasten its end, I should not be able to live with myself now. I should be not only broken in heart by that tragedy, but crucified with remorse.

My personal struggle with the social

services is another story, and that of many such mothers. Few people understand the burden of a handicapped child on the average family, let alone one with a single parent. Financially it is a constant drain, bedding and clothing need repeated changing and replacing. Transport costs money, as does help with housework and shopping, which does not do itself. Where there are other children, a woman is perpetually torn, trying to do justice to all. She cannot go out to work, to keep herself, so has to live on Social Security, and her living standard is forced below subsistence level. She works 24 hours a day, seven days a week, 365 days a year, and has to beg for essentials. Resort to charity and local authority brings the means test. Her name and circumstances are public property. Her home is open to a constant stream of strangers and officials. This not only adds to her own mental and emotional misery, but robs the family of essential privacy. There is now, thanks to the Disablement Income Group, a weekly allowance for families where a patient needs full time attention. Martin did qualify for it, but died before it came into operation. There is no such allowance for a woman whose healthy children also need full time attention. That struggle goes on.

All the pressure from social workers, and the suggested solution for such tragedies as mine, is to put the sick child into an institution. This is sheer cruelty. Home and family are the ideal 'institution' for anyone ill or handicapped, and surely the birthright of any child. For the mother, too, it is agony to have strangers doing what everything in her cries out to do, by her very nature as a mother. I am very grateful for the fact that, where Martin did have outside treatment, I didn't have to pay. But the price of the other side of that coin is a nightmare I would forget if I could.

This society is simply not geared to a mother who wants to give of the utmost to her child. Time and time again, we were forced apart when we needed each other most. We desperately needed money, but as I was receiving a 'pension', I was not allowed to keep what I earned. Every attempt I made to relieve our desperate situation died on a desk, was defeated by a local regulation, or turned down by someone in authority a hundred miles away who had never even met us. My struggle to make a home and keep my family together was not helped, but was positively impeded and obstructed by officials, or the empowerered opinons of State-authorised people. We didn't fit into an appropriate pigeon-hole. There was no specified provision for the likes of me. At the height of our crisis, I did not 'qualify' for a home help. New buildings and a city fly-over are more important than the relief of human suffering. Bureaucracy does not recognise the therapy of love, the sanctity of family, and the basic human right of every individual to die at home. It does not see homes, and the mental peace therein, as fundamental to the structure of a nation. For all this I find it very difficult to take any pride in our Welfare State.

What saved us was the little people: the army of real persons either alone or in voluntary groups and societies, religious orders churches who were moved by our sheer human need, and inspired to meet it, out of the good in their hearts. God used them, as he has to use somebody human, to keep my faith in him and in his Providence alive.

What I owe to my own Catholic Faith is simple. I could not have lived without it. I still believe in miracles. A man whom wind and waves obeyed could very well have shrivelled a tumour, *and* disposed of secondaries. He chose otherwise. In estimating the miraculous, let us not ignore the obvious, the fact that I was able to be with Martin to the very end. He was not my only sorrow, by any means. There were others equally heavy. I had no money and no home. I was alone; stranded in a society where a woman in trouble arouses more hostility than sympathy. I was not in good health, after years of overwork. When I try to tell people the full truth of all that burdened me through that period, they think it impossible. It defies belief. I'm suspected of exaggeration, hysteria, imagination, of lying even. How could one woman do so much? I lived it, and I did it. It happened. It can be verified. There are witnesses. The strains on my mind were enough to drive any sensitive, intelligent woman insane. I gave my mind to God, and he saved it. By the grace of God, we lived, with no permanent damage anywhere.

I am indebted to my 'present moment' way of living, inculcated in me from childhood. Absolute dependence on God, trusting God, leaving all the major issues to him. Concentrating on the here and now, giving all that you've got, never worrying unduly about tomorrow to the extent of getting emotionally involved in its anxieties. It takes great mental discipline, but bears fruit in a courage and patience I found invaluable. Only when God was making a change, did he let me really run down and feel my human frailty.

With Martin, too, I was immensely

grateful for his early religious training. He was fortunate in wonderful schools, in this respect, and God-loving teachers. I couldn't possibly have done at home what they did in his school hours. All I did was confirm and live what he learned away from me. When the time came for him to need his Faith, he was educated to it and prepared. It was all I had to give him. I couldn't have done what I did without his utter abandonment to me, and all I was doing with him: his immediate acceptance of any explanation I gave. He trusted me. I trusted God. Perfect teamwork.

In Martin, in fact, there *was* a miracle. All his nature was against what he had to live. He was not equipped for it. What he learned, day by day, and what he achieved, came from some power inside himself that brought about a complete change. From a sensitive, shy boy who resented even the slightest discomfort, and grumbled at every fault, he turned into one whose afflictions have terrified many an adult, but never complained or felt sorry for himself.

I had to witness his gradual dying to himself, and my strength was not in books, or advice, or secular theories, but in a Woman, also a mother, who had to stand watching her own Son tortured to death for a crime he did not commit. She, too, was alone. She was tough enough to take the truth. I wasn't. But like her, I surrendered my son willingly to God's will, and let him play out the final act himself.

From my Christian Faith I learned the ideal of motherhood, patterned on that Mother and a million lesser women trained to heroism. The fact that I as a nurse is not all that important. I have talked to other women in the same tragic position, and they, too, became what their children needed. They knew by instinct what to do. God gives to mothers, the gift of wisdom where their dependents are concerned. They have to sacrifice a great deal to *be* mothers, and this is their reward. In estimating the miraculous, let us not overlook the supernatural, often super-human quality of motherlove.

I'm indebted to churches, open longer hours than the Ever-open store, and to that familiar miracle that is Communion; water of restoration, source of very real strength and hope. I treasure my capacity for prayer, that often had such dramatic results, that was the escape, so often, of a mind which life had in an iron prison. Under pressure, I opened up into another dimension, where others hold back until it explodes inside.

Death, too, is easier for a mind given to God. Faith sustains and shock is cushioned. There is a reason, always. Looking back, for all my upper conviction that Martin was getting well again, I was at the same time being trained to a sense of loss. Death is easier in a home where children treat it as naturally as birth, and don't get upset about where, or to whom, a brother is gone.

I still believe in Lourdes; that plateau of peace, that State of grace, that retreat without walls. It was a prize deceit, what happened at the Grotto, but it was the only solution. I had to believe in what I was doing. She did to me what I did to Martin. A Mother's guile. Lourdes was the foundation of my ability to cope. In Lourdes I was given a way to look on the face of death and not be afraid. Going back again, without Martin, will be an act of faith calling on more resources than I feel, but emotion never was any guide to what we can achieve. She has already taught me the greatest lesson of all; how to take 'no' for an answer.

I still believe in God, as Father loving and provident; an intelligence beyond human comprehension, more complicated than the most up-to-date machinery, and yet so simple even I can understand. God is love. He gave me all I have. I am all he made me. He has the absolute right to use me, and to take back what he loaned, at any time. For anyone to believe that he does not exist, or does not love, is to me utter ignorance. It is the empty negative to my full positive. They have no experience of him, that's all. That relationship, for me, is constant, inescapable, eternal; above and beyond anything human. I have evidence. Time and again I went to him in torment, and came away at peace. 'Be still and know that I am God.' Somebody bigger and more powerful than any human knew exactly what he was ding. Times I felt ill-treated, abandoned, rejected and ignored. But always by a Person, not a vacuum. He was still there.

He gave us his Son, to teach us how to live, and love, to suffer and to die. My son, too, was crucified. I stayed with the cross, and God let me into his mind. I saw the march of sanctity. I saw the active striving after virtue, then, as God took control, the boy became passive and accepting, perfectly abandoned. God showed me the making of a saint: a super-human.

To some, religion is a combination of mystery and misery; a list of regulations and a rigid, narrow code. To me, it is a fuller, richer form of living; a more expansive outlook, a more, not less, liberal approach. To us, in our human torment, it was what it ought to be; salvation. At every turn, when life failed or trapped us, God set us free. We were saved. He uses suffering; he allows suffering, he never causes it without reason. In that crucible is our purification, our boiling out of defect that can keep us from being happy, here and ever after. He knows what the final end can be, and will pursue it with relentless zeal, for our ultimate joy and thanksgiving. God is not inhuman. Man is inhuman. Man will cause suffering, deliberately, out of a sense of power or to satisfy something in himself. When it comes to mercy, God is quicker. There are humans who have none at all.

In Martin's life, God gave me quality, not quantity. I gave up my life to him, and he gave his for me. When life offers you a cross, you can either cling or run. We clung together. It is not the way of the world, the hallmark of which is to avoid suffering by any means. We live in a society where many women spend more time looking after themselves, machines and animals than other humans. It is taken for granted a woman will wish to avoid what is hard, unpleasant and difficult, and that motherhood will take second place to her own interest. So when she sees motherhood as her divine calling, along with necessary vows of poverty, chastity and obedience, and she actually *wants* to crucify herself for her young, she is widely despised, reviled, despaired of and generally misunderstood. She is pensioned off by the State, deprived of human status and dignity, treated with official apathy and social disdain. She is made to feel a parasite and a dropout and no use on earth because all she does is stay at home and look after children. Her earning power is nil.

All this I lived, and suffered, and did not relish, but it taught me a very great deal. It showed me what power can do in the hands of the immature. It forced me to see men worshipping false gods of systems, money, snobbery, ambition and books of rules; making living sacrifices of human minds and lives upon their altars. It gave me a perception of wickedness in the modern world that I often wish I had been spared. It gave me the courage to face up to big people, and realise how very small they are after all.

Suffering is like a woman in labour. It comes in waves. Under God, with his purpose in mind, there is a lesson in each session. It is always productive; never wasted. Mine was a rich experience, and one I am glad to have lived through. I have known a great love that nobody can take from me, though there are those who would. Spiritual envy is a prevalent evil still.

I have said goodbye to Martin's body, but not his mind, or his will to be with me, and relieve me. His suffering is over. He will never suffer again. He can never be killed in a war, away from me, or tortured at the hands of aliens. He can never turn his back on God and deny the Faith we lived by. He is safe. There are so many ways a mother can lose a son. It comforts me that he never lost his innocence; that pure essence so derided today. That is no mean achievement in an overstimulated generation fed sophistication from the cot. Children today are given sex and poison drugs to play with while still at school. And adults encourage them—call it 'freedom'. He is spared that, and I feel relief. He is a clean memory.

Death is not the end of life, but a change of lives. The dead are not without intelligence, nor yet are they asleep. Their reason is their driving force, and the good, or those who have at last achieved a stage of *wanting* to be good, are extremely happy, and they are free. That love survives the grave, and can maintain a new relationship, is a fact, and a reality.

Martin won the martyr's crown, as surely as many a Christian before him. Of the destination of a child of that age and perfection of character there can be no doubt. It scares me not a little just how much one person has to suffer to be rendered perfect in God's sight, and fit for Paradise. I have never yet prayed *for* Martin, only to him. For him I lost my human dignity, but he has in his turn raised me. I am the mother of a saint, who has great pulling power with God, and will surely save us, as a family. My first anguished prayer to him was not given an immediate 'yes', or not to my knowledge anyway. But I accept that the mark of a saint, in Heaven as on earth, is submission to the will and purpose of God. I still believe. I go on, hoping.

Days when faith is high and life light, I think of his cheeky wit and brave smile and chirpy ingenuity. He's a happy thought. I feel his impish spirit at my elbow. Days when I am heavy with stress and pregnant with grief on other crosses, I'd willingly relinquish my life here to be with him again. His tower of manly sanctity is gone from me, and I need it so. I cling to his brothers and sisters, but not too hard. It would not be fair to them. I think they have forgotten, till one of them says, 'It's not the same without Martin is it?' We are a wounded community. One day it will be healed, leaving only a scar. Always he will be one of us. In every difficulty, every need, we turn as of habit, to our little patron in

Paradise, and in no time see the benefit.

Why couldn't he have lived? Because he was born in an age in which cancer is the biggest killer of our nation's children, and life conspired to accelerate a potential with which he was born. There are those who will think he ought not to have been born. All I can say is, 'Ask Martin'. He knows the whole story. He is the only one qualified to judge whether it was worth it.

Now his story is told, as I saw it, and I lived it with him. My last task for him is done. It has made me suffer, sometimes unbearably. A dozen times I have set it aside, promising myself 'I will not *do* it.' And always, after a little rest, that little voice prompted me, 'Get on with the book.' He is as set on my purification as God was on his, and would not let me be. Now it is done, and the hardest, heaviest blow to accept is how much he need not have suffered, how much we both could have been spared, and even whether, had things been more humane and geared to our sad circumstances, he would have died at all.

He was born of a bitterly unhappy marriage, with no real parental unity. Founding a family on a fractured base is no easy undertaking and I was coming to the end of my strength on that account. Keeping domestic harmony in the presence, night and day, of a destructive adult relationship, gradually nearing physical violence, is like living on a precipice. Yet Martin was not unhappy, until the tensions could no longer be kept from harming him, and all of us. Then I had to leave. I tried to make a new home for my children; a safe, happier, more secure Christian community, based on my own religious life. I was on all sides opposed, slandered, criticised and condemned. I was branded 'deserter' and put under pressure to go back on my conscientious decision, worked out over harrowing months, before God, on my knees. I was made a pauper, forced to feel I had violated every code of human decency. But out of confusion came conviction. There again, I know I did the right thing.

And there again, it was people who had never lived my particular agony who had the most to say. They isolated and rejected me when I needed friendly support. They assumed they knew the will of God for me, in their utter ignorance of my private life and domestic responsibility. I pray the strength to forgive. They punished an innocent child for what *they*saw as a crime and a spiritual felony. They know not what they do.

My own Church, with the power and authority endowed to it by God, has recognised my private conscience, respected my decision, blessed my home and counted us a worthy part of its community. That will suffice for me. I am free, under God and the State, to worship as I please, and to bring up my children in the Faith that is their heritage. There are those who would deny me that freedom, but disillusion over human nature is a part of facing truth. I accept that reality too.

Ours is a success story, because we took on insuperable odds, and we overcame them. We did the impossible. The tumour is dead. Martin lives. Ours is the victory.